Leslie Sansone's

Eat Smart, Walk Strong

The Secrets to Effortless Weight Loss

Leslie Sansone

Recipes by Rowan Jacobsen

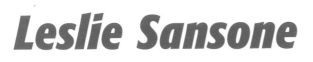

CENTER STREET™

NEW YORK   BOSTON   NASHVILLE

Publisher's Note: This book is not intended to replace a one-on-one relationship with a qualified health-care professional and is not intended as medical advice, but as a sharing of knowledge and information from the research and experience of the author. You are advised and encouraged to consult with your health-care professional in all matters relating to your health.

Center Street
Hachette Book Group USA
1271 Avenue of the Americas, New York, NY 10020
Visit our Web site at www.centerstreet.com

Printed in the United States of America
Originally published in hardcover by Center Street
Center Street is a division of Hachette Book Group USA. The Center Street name and logo are trademarks of Hachette Book Group USA.
First Trade Edition: January 2007
10 9 8 7 6 5 4 3 2 1

The Library of Congress has cataloged the hardcover edition as follows:

Sansone, Leslie.
  (Eat Smart, walk strong)
  Leslie Sansone's eat smart, walk strong : the secrets to effortless weight loss / Leslie Sansone.
       p. cm.
  ISBN 1-931722-51-X
1. Fitness walking. 2. Weight loss. 3. Reducing exercises. I. Title.

RA781.65.S22 2006
613.7--dc22

                                                                2005022162

Book designed by Mada Design, Inc.
ISBN 10: 0-446-69337-5(pbk.)
ISBN 13: 987-0-446-69337-0(pbk.)

CONTENTS

You Can Enjoy Life to Its Fullest

Congratulations on your commitment to improve your health, your vitality, and your life. By choosing to read this book, you have taken the first step toward achieving a better life. Good health is an investment that pays enormous dividends in personal energy, emotional health, and even relationships.

It's possible you picked up this book today because you're frustrated by your current weight or health condition. Maybe you've tried to lose weight in the past but had little or no success. The thought of beginning this journey again may seem overwhelming. If so, let me take a moment to encourage you.

I have been a nutritionist deeply committed to public health for over twenty years. As head of the Center of Nutritional Excellence at Florida Hospital, I have talked to numerous people who are confused by all the conflicting information available today about weight loss and healthy eating. I have counseled thousands of people and seen countless individuals make astonishing improvements in weight loss and physical conditions. No matter what your previous health history, you *can* begin a new chapter today.

That's why I'm so pleased to introduce Leslie Sansone's new book, *Eat Smart, Walk Strong*. In these pages, Leslie does an amazing job of cutting through the hype surrounding healthy weight loss and gets to the heart of the matter. Her message is simple: Small healthy changes can make a big difference. You don't have to give up all your favorite foods or start running marathons to achieve healthy weight loss. But, like most Americans, you probably need to make *some* small changes, which will reap great benefits.

As a registered dietitian, I love the title Leslie chose for this book. It describes the passion to which I have dedicated my life—teaching people how to eat for optimal health. Leslie does not push people toward extremes; her approach is sensible. Success is not about restriction as much as it is about moderation and balance. In that respect, Leslie's recommendations are eminently doable.

Perhaps the thing I admire most about Leslie is the way she lives what she believes. Not only does she keep herself trim and fit, but she has proven her commitment to healthy living through her wildly popular *Walk Away the Pounds* book and video series. Leslie's greatest achievement, however, may be the way she makes healthy living pleasurable. Most of us don't like to exercise. So Leslie shows us how to make it fun. Many of us don't enjoy eating healthy foods. Leslie shows us how to make it a delight.

Americans in general are an overfed society. Yet for many people, the pleasure has gone out of eating. How can this be? Today, many people eat because they are bored, sad, worried, frustrated, or angry. They use food as a stress reliever, not to alleviate hunger. Others are in such a rush from busy schedules that they have little time to eat, so they wolf down something that's fast and convenient before running off to their next activity. These eating extremes rob food of the simple pleasure it can bring us. They can also lead to overeating, indigestion, and a host of bad habits. We need to put the simple enjoyment of eating back into our lives. Leslie encourages us to do just that! She shows us how to regain the pleasure in eating good food that will make us look and feel great.

In my work as a nutritionist, I advise my patients to do three things. First, make a decision to change. Second, set realistic goals and create an action plan. Third, find a partner or group of people who will support you. These three steps are crucial to your long-term success. That's why I'm so pleased with Leslie's six-week plan. Here you will find the encouragement you need to make a positive change. That's step one. You will also find a workable action plan that will help you reach your goals. That's step two. To achieve step three, I recommend you find yourself a partner, buy that person a copy of this book, and go through it together. Better yet, get a group from your work, school, neighborhood, health club, church, or circle of family and friends to join you. You will greatly increase your chances of reaching your weight-loss goal and attaining success.

Leslie Sansone's Eat Smart, Walk Strong is not merely about weight loss. It's about adopting powerful strategies and forming healthy habits that will help you enjoy life to its fullest. I applaud you and respect you for taking action to give yourself and those you love the most valuable gift of extraordinary health. You have the ability to create a better, healthier life. Don't wait; start today. Follow the plan outlined in these pages and you will learn to eat smart, walk strong, and live life to its fullest.

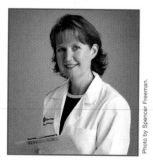

Photo by Spencer Freeman.

Sherri Flynt, MPH, RD, LD
Author, speaker, counselor
Head of the Center of Nutritional Excellence,
Florida Hospital, Orlando (the largest hospital in America)

Who Is This Book For?

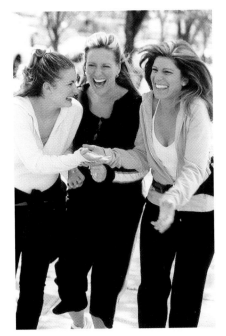

All of us, large and small, old and young, male and female, have certain eating patterns we'd like to improve. That's why I designed this book to focus on more than just weight loss. The healthy lifestyle strategies I use will bring about weight loss if you are overweight, but they'll also improve the energy and cardiovascular health of naturally slender people. No matter what your goals are, you will find that adopting these new habits makes life easier, less stressful, and more fun.

I hope you'll give my program a try no matter who you are. You may be one of the many people who will find this program a godsend, especially if you fit any of these descriptions:

- You used my first book but find you still struggle sometimes with your eating choices.
- You work out with my videos and want structure for the eating half of the weight-loss equation.
- You've never heard of me in your life, but know you aren't eating as well as you should and want some tips that will easily fit into your day.
- You get hours of exercise every week but still can't seem to lose those last ten pounds.
- You're tired of denying yourself all the off-limit foods on the low-carb diets and want a program that delivers the same weight loss with greater flexibility.
- You have a good idea what your needs are and want a program you can customize to work with your strengths.
- You're sick of self-help books telling you that your diet dilemma stems from deep character flaws or self-esteem issues, when you know it has a lot more to do with the fact that ice cream tastes really, really good.
- You've tried to lose weight through willpower alone and have discovered that willpower is the first thing to desert people when the going gets tough.

- You are very good at eating well, staying active, and losing weight on vacation, but you find that when day-to-day life returns, so do the bad habits.
- You don't take dieting too seriously but would love to get in shape and lose a few pounds if this would require no extra work on your part.

Ring any bells? If so, then you are going to love my food plan! It's easy to learn, fun to follow, and flexible enough to give you whatever you need at this moment in your life. So you have nothing to lose. If you know me, you know I wouldn't have it any other way.

Who Is This Book Not For?

If you are looking for a weight-loss shortcut, then this isn't the book for you. There are no shortcuts to lasting weight loss, and don't believe anyone who tells you otherwise. On the other hand, weight loss isn't hard; it just requires a steady commitment from you. The most important component of losing weight is *staying active*. That's right, I'm talking about exercise! Exercise, especially walking, is the long-term key to fitness and weight control.

In this book, I assume that you are already on an exercise walking plan or are ready to start one. (If not, read chapter 4, "Exercise: The Most Important Nutrient," and you'll be ready!) I also include a box on each day of your six-week journal in which to record your exercise. You'll find that the weight-loss benefits of eating right really kick in when accompanied by a daily walk.

Some people like a full-fledged diet plan that spells out what to eat for every meal and includes complete nutritional information with all recipes. This isn't that kind of book. Such diet plans already exist, and they work well for some people. For example, I've known lots of women who have used my walking program in conjunction with the food plans offered by Jenny Craig, Weight Watchers, or TOPS. They've had good results! I'm not a doctor or a licensed nutritionist, and I don't pretend to offer a food plan as thorough or comprehensive as those just mentioned. If that's what you think you need, I encourage you to seek them out. If, however, you are looking for simple common sense to help you jettison some bad old habits and effortlessly develop good new ones, then you've come to the right place. **Welcome!**

PART I

WE MAKE OUR HABITS, AND THEN THEY MAKE US

1. Learning to Love Food Again

Have I got some good news for you! Over the past few years, we have seen revolutions in both the science of nutrition and the development of weight-loss strategies, and those revolutions are going to make our lives a lot better. After decades of fad diets and bum science, we have finally reached a point where we know that eating fat won't necessarily make us fat and starving ourselves won't make us slim. We know that commonsense eating and an active lifestyle are what keep us fit and beautiful, and that few foods are "off the table" when it comes to planning a diet. With this knowledge, you can customize your own weight-loss plan— one that is easier, more flexible, and more effective than you ever imagined possible—and this book will show you how.

I want to help you make food a more delicious and exciting part of your life. I know that sounds strange for a weight-loss book. But this isn't any ordinary book. After hearing from so many fans of my walking book and videos who struggle with overeating, I realized there is a fundamental problem with many food diets. They are about rejection, about denying yourself enjoyment. And that is a very tough row to hoe. I thought about what methods I use to keep myself eating sensibly, and I realized that the secret is learning to love food more, to approach it with reverence and celebration. Anything approached with reverence is less likely to be abused.

Think about the act of saying grace before a meal. Partly this is to give thanks to God for providing the food, but it also serves to get our attention, to make us more conscious of the goodness of the food. I even think it makes food taste better. And I believe this act of developing a more intentional relationship with food—loving it, savoring it, and not taking it for granted—can actually make us eat less and enjoy it more.

We like to think that we already eat intentionally. Unfortunately, most of us are in a lot less control than we'd like to be, even those making a concerted effort to diet. Tell me if this scenario sounds familiar.

You did the weekly shopping a couple of days ago and loaded up on healthy food, straight out of the low-carb diet book you've been reading. Tonight, you'll make chicken breasts with sun-dried tomatoes and broccoli on the side, plus a salad. A healthy meal for the whole family!

Despite your best intentions, though, things don't go as planned. You run a little late at work. By the time you get home, it's nearly six o'clock. The kids are starving. *You're* starving. Everyone needs a nibble while you start dinner. What's ready to go? Chips. Maybe cheese and crackers or honey-roasted peanuts. Within minutes, an entire tub of peanuts and a two-liter bottle of Coke have disappeared while you pulled ingredients out of the fridge.

Now it's almost 6:30 and you've got to bake chicken breasts; wash, chop, and steam broccoli; dice sun-dried tomatoes; and so on. You're looking at an hour until dinner. And your son has a basketball game in thirty minutes. Even the prospect of washing and spinning the lettuce seems like a pain.

On the other hand, there are two frozen sausage pizzas in the freezer that can be ready in ten minutes. You know which choice your husband would prefer.

Problem solved.

Except, this is actually problem created. Even though you made perfectly rational decisions—you had to tie things up at work before leaving, you were too pooped to make a whole meal, and you had to get *something* in your son before he disappeared—the result is that you and your family wound up eating a meal that contributes to weight gain, diabetes, heart disease, and other problems.

This is just one example of the many compromises we make and habits we fall into in the course of our daily lives. None of these choices seems especially terrible in itself, but taken together, over the course of years, they add up to an obesity epidemic.

No amount of knowing that we should choose the salmon and brown rice over the burger and fries is going to solve this, because it isn't a question of knowledge or intentions. There are times in our lives when we are on the ball, when we have an extra hour and use it to create a beautiful, nurturing meal for the whole family, or when we order the grilled chicken salad in a restaurant and manage to escape without succumbing to dessert or scarfing down the entire basket of rolls. When our energy is good, we're all capable of making good food decisions. The slips happen when we're tired, starving, rushed, or simply overwhelmed by temptation. Those moments are going to happen to all of us from time to time. The trick is to learn to head them off at the pass whenever possible, and to have healthier, *equally convenient* solutions at hand when those moments do strike.

When our energy is good, we're all capable of making good food decisions. The slips happen when we're tired, starving, rushed, or simply overwhelmed by temptation.

Learning such tricks and strategies is what this book is all about. What makes this program such an exciting departure from traditional weight-loss books is that it will help you develop smart eating habits that become second nature, where eating healthy food requires no more effort or willpower from you than choosing junk food did. The low-carb diets (or even the old low-fat diets, for that matter) work great, *if you can stick to them*. How many people do you know who started a low-carb diet, lost real weight, and looked great but then a year later wound up right back where they'd started? I know quite a few. From them, I realized that to start solving America's weight problem, we needed to stop focusing on *what* people should be eating and instead focus on *why* they eat unhealthily in the first place.

Behavioral psychologists have been studying people's eating habits for some time. The things they've found may sound all too familiar. For instance:

- Convenience is a major factor in what people choose to eat. Having to cook is a drawback.
- Access is key. If candy is within arm's reach, it is hard to resist. If it is out of sight in a cupboard, we eat less of it. If it isn't in the house at all, we are very unlikely to actually get in the car and seek it out.
- The main causes of overeating bouts are not hunger or the deliciousness of the food, but emotional and psychological cravings.
- Larger serving sizes make us consume more food (even if we don't finish the serving).
- There is little relationship between meals; for example, eating a large lunch will not help us eat a small dinner.

- We eat or drink more from large half-filled containers than from small full ones but believe we have consumed less.
- We are more susceptible to suggestion than we think.

This is just the tip of the iceberg. In presenting the six-week food plan, I'll explain the many mind games we play on ourselves (and food companies play on us), and I'll give you the tools you need to deprogram yourself. The best thing about these findings is that they make for some of the easiest fixes imaginable! Forget the idea that seemingly insurmountable problems require heroic solutions. I've spent my career teaching people that the solution to their exercise and weight challenges lies in taking simple steps that develop into an ongoing habit. Food issues are no different. As you repeat these small changes in your habits, you'll find that, like a seesaw, momentum suddenly swings to the other side and everything happens on its own. You just have to hold on for the ride, which is why you are going to find my Eat Smart, Walk Strong plan the easiest, most effective program you have ever tried, and you are going to have fun doing it!

If you've done Walk Diets with me in the past, you're going to enjoy this variation. It's still a six-week program, but this time the amount of walking you do stays the same (the amount is up to you), while your diet gets healthier and healthier. That makes this plan ideal for people who have reached a level of exercise they like but who still want to lose more weight.

How can changing a lifetime of eating habits be fun, or easy? I'm glad you asked! So many reasons jump to mind. Here are some of my favorites:

- **A whole new relationship with food.** For many of us, food is a burden as much as a comfort. We love food, but we struggle with the temptations and the guilt, the way it makes us feel bad about ourselves. Having to count calories takes away the enjoyment of eating and turns it into a math game fraught with worry. That's why you don't count calories on my Eat Smart, Walk Strong plan. Instead, you cultivate smart lifestyle habits that help you exercise naturally and eat right *without* thinking so hard about it.
- **More flexibility.** Many diets have a one-size-fits-all mentality. But we all have different tastes and different factors influencing our lives, and the solution to anyone's diet dilemma is going to be unique to that person. My PERFECT Support System is designed to flex each week as you customize it to work with you, not in spite of you.
- **Discovering delicious new foods.** We all tend to develop eating ruts, where the same twenty foods rotate through our meals each week. By venturing into some new areas and trying some unique yet easy recipes, you'll get a lot more variety and enjoyment in your diet.

- **Better energy and mood.** It's amazing how a poor diet can sap my energy. I feel sleepy, sluggish, uncreative, and foggy. Then, when I start eating right, the fog lifts. I practically leap into my walking routine, and tasks like everyday problem solving—or even finding the energy to cook—seem to come quite easily. I get more accomplished and my emotions stay on an even keel.
- **Better health.** There are few things more frustrating than having an illness or condition that prevents you from trying new things or participating in certain activities. Eating right is your best medicine; it will ensure a lifetime of fun with friends and family, instead of hours spent worrying about your body.
- **Better looks.** You are what you eat, and guess what? You look like what you eat, too! It's easy to see the difference between healthy eaters and unhealthy ones by looking at their bodies, faces, and skin. And we all know that looking better makes us feel better about ourselves, and feeling better keeps us a lot more active, engaged, and content.
- **Better spirit.** As I said at the beginning, food is one of our most direct ways of connecting with the source of all life. Stay connected to that source and everything else falls into place.

Together, you and I are going to make all these things happen in your life. Our secret is pattern-busting activities we use to break you out of old habits and into healthy new ones. These activities may be powerful, but they aren't hard. They involve actions as simple as turning off the TV while you eat, reinventing breakfast, and choosing glasses and dishes that reinforce your eating goals. If you can do those things, you can change the way you eat and the way you live.

Remember to take this one step at a time. I've laid it all out for you. Each day for six weeks, just flip open to the page for that day and follow the plan. By the end of the six weeks, you'll have established a team of good habits that will serve as your personal motivation coach, trainer, and Secret Service agents to keep you on course and prevent destructive behaviors from getting anywhere near you.

This program is going to have a sensational impact on your waistline, but I hope it goes further than that. I know how lonely and isolating it can be when food becomes a trouble spot in your life. But I also know the pleasure that comes from preparing wholesome food and sharing it with family and friends. Eating is a spiritual act. Let's get started on rediscovering that spirit.

TEN EASY LIFESTYLE CHANGES TO IMPROVE YOUR HEALTH

Daily Change	Result	Tips for Forming Habit
30-minute walk	Lose 20 pounds in one year Cut risk of diabetes by 58% Cut risk of heart disease by 45%	Chapter 4
Replace 1 tablespoon butter with olive oil	Cut risk of heart attack by 50%	Chapter 9
Replace 1 soda/juice with water	Lose 10 pounds in one year	Chapter 7
Replace meat twice per week with fish	Lose 10 pounds in one year Cut risk of heart attack by 40%	Chapter 12
Replace white rice, potatoes, and white bread with whole grains	Cut risk of heart disease by 30% Cut risk of diabetes by 30%	Chapter 8
Stop eating transfats˙	Cut risk of heart disease by 50%	Chapter 9
Reduce diet by 100 calories	Lose 10 pounds in one year	Chapters 7, 9
5 servings of fruits and veggies	Cut risk of heart attack by 15% Cut risk of stroke by 30% Cut risk of many cancers	Chapters 10, 11
Drink 8 cold glasses of water	Lose 10 pounds in one year	Chapter 7
Stop smoking	Cut risk of cancer by 30% Cut risk of heart disease by 50%	
OVERALL	Lose 60 pounds in one year Cut risk of early death by 80%	

Found in margarine, crackers, chips, fast food, nondairy creamer, cake mixes, some peanut butter, and packaged cakes, cookies, doughnuts, and pies.

2. The PERFECT Support System

I love habits! Having a collection of good habits is like being the head of a company of highly skilled employees who do their jobs without needing constant management. The company runs itself, leaving you free to make the big decisions. That's what your life should be like. If you need to act like a micromanager over your life, constantly using willpower to overrule your natural impulses, you are going to be exhausted, and you aren't going to have much success anyway. You are the boss of your life, and the time has come for a company shake-up.

You can't just fire your bad habits, though. They won't leave! They're like ex-employees clinging to their desks while the security team yanks on their ankles. No, when it comes to habits, you have to bring in the new habits— the star employees who are going to make you a wild success— and give them all the responsibility. Pretty soon, the old habits have nothing left to do and disappear on their own! You'll discover how incredibly easy it is to succeed when you have the right habits working for you. You'll learn the secrets of those naturally fit people who never seem tempted by the bloomin' onion, who always find time for a walk, who have tons of energy, and who stay slim without dieting. In fact, I'll tell you some of their secrets right now: They *aren't* tempted by the deep-fried onion (because they've trained their bodies to crave foods that make them feel good), they walk every day because their bodies are used to it and get an urge to do it as surely as some people get an urge for chocolate, they have tons of energy because they exercise and eat high-energy food, and they stay slim because they *don't* crash-diet, but instead keep their metabolisms high by eating plenty of healthy foods.

None of these healthy behaviors takes an ounce of extra willpower or concentration. The reason some people make it look so easy is because *it really is that easy*. However they first got started, they repeated these positive behaviors long enough to turn them into habits. As we all know, good or bad, habits are very hard to break.

Your task, as I said before, is to develop healthy, effective new habits that will squeeze out those old habits you don't like. The way to achieve this is by taking small steps every day. You don't need to make any drastic changes, as long as you keep your eyes fixed on the horizon and your long-term goals. Keep those goals in

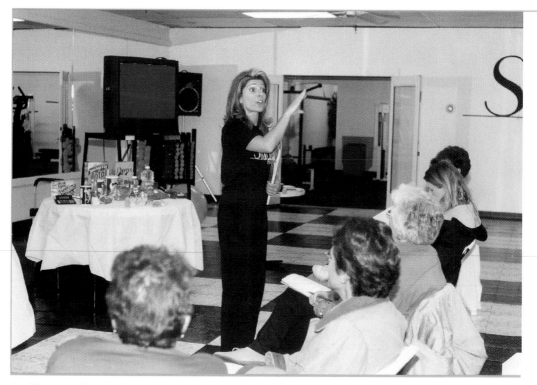

Teaching a nutrition class at Studio Fitness. We try to give our members everything they need for healthy living.

sight, keep getting one step closer to them, and before you know it, you will be one of those people others marvel at for making it look so easy.

Let me introduce you to your assistant in this endeavor. It's called the PERFECT Support System. Think of it as your ticket to a perfect life! That doesn't mean you'll be rich, famous, and will achieve world peace, but it will help you attain what I see as a perfect life: good health, a great self-image, richly fulfilling days, and the chance to accomplish anything you want.

The PERFECT Support System has seven keys to success:

Plan your good habits.

Educate yourself about which behaviors keep you healthy and slim.

Repeat your new behaviors until they become habits.

Flex your plan to customize it to your needs, desires, and personal tastes.

Exercise to stay trim and energized.

Celebrate your new life to keep your spirit involved.

Transform into the person you always wanted to be.

Let's look at each step more closely.

1. PLAN

As I said earlier, we're all capable of making good eating decisions when good choices are available to us, off-limits temptations aren't, and time isn't a factor. The key to making those positive situations happen is *planning ahead* by identifying the things that trip us up and going into the upcoming week with a specific game plan for giving ourselves the best chance of success. A page at the end of each week will help you do so.

2. EDUCATE YOURSELF

All the education you need to lose permanent weight is right here in this book. At least I can take care of that much for you! Each week of the six-week food plan introduces one eating habit that can help you lose weight effortlessly. You may already have some of these habits mastered. If so, don't worry about it; you'll have an easy week!

Along with a healthy habit, each week introduces one type of food that can help keep you less hungry and more fulfilled. Each day during the week (except Sunday, your day off) includes a tip for implementing the new habit and some recipe suggestions for trying out the new food.

By the end of the six weeks, you'll be an expert on nutrition and smart living. You'll know how to keep your family fueled on good food and how to recognize growing behavior traps so you can nip them in the bud.

3. REPEAT HEALTHY BEHAVIORS

Once you learn these keys to healthy living, you need to keep doing them. Repeating behaviors establishes new habits. The time required to establish a new habit varies with the activity and the person, but experts consider twenty-one days to be the general rule. Do something every day for twenty-one days, and you will keep doing it. Your brain actually changes physically! New pathways develop in your neurons, muscle memory takes hold, and it becomes harder to stop the behavior than to keep doing it. That's what a habit is.

By the end of this six-week program, you'll have repeated your healthy behaviors enough to make them a natural part of your life. You've got new habits! By then, you'll be seeing impressive differences in your waistline, your energy level, and your attitude. After that, maintaining those habits is the name of the game.

4. FLEX THE PLAN TO SUIT YOUR NEEDS

We'll spend a lot of time in this book focusing on both familiar and surprising reasons why people get trapped in bad eating habits, but you can probably identify a few of your own already. The Flex Questionnaire on page 36 will help clarify which particular eating issues give you trouble. Those are the ones to work on the hardest. More likely than not, they can be fixed by changing the patterns in your day-to-day life that set you up for failure.

The tips and recipes in the six-week program are extremely easy to follow—the goal is to make your life easier, after all—but don't worry, you aren't expected to follow them all. Life just doesn't work that way. Some will fit smoothly into your life; some, for whatever reason, won't. That's fine. This plan is flexible enough to change your life without derailing it. Too many diets fail because they treat people as if they all have the same likes and dislikes—and we know that's not the case. For some people, eating the right foods at breakfast can change the entire dynamic of how they eat during the day, preventing the blood-sugar extremes that cause hunger attacks and panicky eating. For others, having convenient, ready-to-eat veggies on hand is the key to squelching the junk-food habit.

That's why I give you many options each week for ways to implement your healthy habit. Skip the suggestions you know won't work in your life, but don't ignore the ones you think will. Flexibility means designing your own program and *committing* yourself, on a daily basis, to following your new behaviors. A page at the end of each week will help you distinguish what worked for you that week, so you can plan your patterns for the upcoming week.

5. EXERCISE

Of all the healthy habits you can establish, none is more important than exercise. Daily walking will deliver as many benefits as all your eating strategies combined. I feel so strongly about this that I made it the focus of my entire first book! Many of you will already be on a walking routine when you undertake this program. If you aren't, please read my chapter on exercise and begin walking as soon as possible.

6. CELEBRATE!

When you reach the end of the six weeks and suddenly *know*, in your heart, that you are truly committed to continuing your new healthy lifestyle, you'll certainly want to celebrate, but I hope you'll start the celebration long before then. No need to throw a big party; I think of celebration as a daily event, a party for you and yourself. Celebrate by giving thanks for your exciting new life and by reminding yourself just how good it feels. This kind of celebration not only keeps you aware of how beneficial your new habits are; it also feels good in and of itself. It makes life richer, and becomes a great positive feedback loop: The better you feel, the more you want to celebrate; the more you celebrate, the better you feel. And there's *always* something worth celebrating in each day—it's just a matter of remembering to look.

7. TRANSFORM

Did you know that your skin cells completely renew themselves every two weeks? And many of the rest of your cells aren't far behind. By the end of these six weeks, you will have truly transformed at every level. All that healthy food will have been used to remodel most cells in your body. You'll be the new, improved You! With high-quality materials, an improved design set up by your new habits, and a clear vision for the future, there will be no stopping you. (This would be a good time to throw that big party!)

There is no particular order to how you should implement these seven keys. They are all ongoing behaviors I hope you'll adopt permanently—even transformation. As you go through the six-week food plan, keep the PERFECT acronym in mind, because it's important not to let any of these behaviors slip. Like the arches, domes, and buttresses of a cathedral, they all reinforce one another; if you take one away, the others are weakened. Stop celebrating each day, for example, and your spirit won't feel invested in your goal. Then the eating and exercise can start to feel like work. Stop exercising, and you'll burn fewer calories each day and will find it difficult to lose weight no matter how well you eat.

But you won't let any of these behaviors slip. How do I know? Well, I do have complete faith in you, but I'll remind you every week, just to make sure. On Sundays, you get a break from your exercise and eating goals. Instead, all you have to do is fill out a wrap-up page, where you track your progress using the PERFECT Support System. It's an easy way of keeping your focus. After two or three weeks of these Sunday wrap-ups, you'll hardly need to fill out these pages to stay on task. You'll do it automatically in your head; staying focused will be just one more good habit you've added to your repertoire!

NEWS YOU CAN USE

If you feel like all your favorite foods are off-limits in your diet, then you are on the wrong diet. We live in exciting nutritional times. Don't believe me? Then look at this list of foods, once off-limits but now known to offer powerful health benefits. Eat them all guilt-free—but in moderation.

Chocolate	**Olive Oil**
Avocados	**Nuts**
Egg	**Wine**

3. The Straight Facts on Nutrition and Weight Loss

There are constant new companies that stand to make a lot of money by confusing you about weight loss. Their hopes of getting you to buy their diet foods and pills rest on convincing you that good nutrition is a complex science, that you'll need experts and special help to achieve weight loss.

The diet-food industry has been abetted by well-meaning scientists searching for the keys to why we gain weight. When these scientists solve one piece of the weight puzzle, the media hypes their discovery, and soon a whole industry forms around that one element. This is what happened with the low-fat craze of the nineties, and it's happening again with the low-carb craze of today.

Some good education came out of both of these diet trends. We're all a lot more savvy about nutrition than we used to be. But too often, focusing on one element of nutrition encourages people to ignore the big picture. People thought all they needed to do was cut fat or carbs, and then they could do anything else they wanted. They weren't being told that the truth about weight loss is incredibly simple. Here it is:

The only way to lose weight is to burn more calories a day than you eat!

Pretty simple, huh? But you can't really sell diet products by telling people that. (Unless you're selling pills that promise to "boost your metabolism." Sorry, the only ways to boost your metabolism are exercise, regular sleep, and healthy eating.) We'd all love a shortcut to weight loss, so we seize on one when it's offered to us. Unfortunately, that allows us to ignore the basics, things like portion size and total calorie intake. **The average woman today eats 335 more calories per day than did the average woman thirty years ago.** That's alarming.

Here's one more number to keep in mind (and after this, I promise, no more math). Every 10 extra calories eaten per day result in 1 pound of weight gain per year. So 335 extra calories per day add up to 33.5 pounds per year. For most of us, those thirty-plus pounds are the whole shebang. If we could eliminate those, we'd be sitting pretty.

The good news? The opposite is true, too. Every 10 calories you cut from your daily diet result in 1 pound of weight loss per year. You can easily shave those

Every 10 calories you cut from your daily diet result in 1 pound of weight loss per year.

thirty-some pounds in a year without eliminating any particular foods or embracing any fad diet. Once you understand the nutrition basics, you'll see why paying attention to *why* you overeat and learning to change your habits will pay off faster than simply cutting certain foods from your diet.

NUTRITION AND ENERGY

Food is energy. It's our only source of fuel, and it provides us with the power we need to do everything we do: to walk, talk, think, breathe, and laugh. It allows us to hug our kids, weed our garden, and run a marathon. It also provides the energy for things our bodies take care of automatically; for example, it keeps our heart beating and our skin replenishing itself.

The energy that food provides is measured in calories. That's also the way we measure the amount of work it takes our bodies to do anything. If you weigh 120 pounds, you use about twelve hundred calories just doing the basics of staying alive: breathing, digesting, talking, walking around your house and office, and sitting or standing upright. If you are larger than this, you burn a little more. If you are more muscular, you also burn more, because muscle uses energy all the time to keep its form, while fat doesn't (fat is your body's energy storage). This basic amount of energy burned is your resting metabolism. Beyond this, you burn calories through physical activity. A brisk half-hour walk burns about two hundred calories. So does an hour of gardening.

Whatever amount of energy we use, we need to make sure we get enough from our food to support those activities. That's not a problem for most of us in America, where food is plentiful. What's more common is getting more calories from food than we need. When that happens, our bodies take the extra, unburned calories and store them as fat.

Don't blame the body. It's just being responsible. If we earn more money than we need to support our lifestyle, we try to store the extra in savings or retirement accounts, knowing that a day will come when we'll need it. The body does the same thing. Before the invention of modern agriculture and transportation, food shortages were common. A body that could draw on that savings account of fat when times got tough was much more likely to survive.

In the modern world, however, most of us never experience tough times foodwise. Still, our bodies act like misers who learned to squirrel away as much as possible and can't stop, even as those bank accounts on our thighs grow fatter than we will ever need. Like a miserly old uncle, they hate to give up even a little of what they've saved.

Fortunately, you can get that uncle to loosen up his checkbook. The more your body gets used to burning calories every day through exercise, the more willing it will be to do so in the future. (And the more it will need to burn to maintain your increased muscle.)

The other side of the equation is the main focus for this book. If we cut the uncle's income down to no more than he needs, he can't squirrel any more away.

The question is: Exactly how much do we need, and of what?

PROTEIN, CARBOHYDRATES, AND FAT

As you've noticed in the nutrition facts found on every food package, food is divided into three main nutrients: protein, carbohydrates, and fat. Despite what certain media reports may have led you to believe, there are no bad nutrients. You need them all! Each plays a different role in the body.

Protein

Protein is the building material of the body. In a way, you are protein. Your muscles and organs are made of protein, as is your skin. Your bones and brain contain protein, too. Protein is pretty important stuff. Your body needs to get enough of it every day to rebuild body tissue, to build new muscle, and to create the hormones, enzymes, immune cells, and other tiny workers that keep the body functioning. You can't store extra protein in your body for a later date, which is why you need a fresh supply daily.

Fortunately, few of us have any trouble finding enough protein. A 140-pound woman needs about 56 grams of protein per day—which is about the amount found in one quarter-pound hamburger or other serving of meat or fish. Animal flesh is primarily protein. Other good sources of protein include dairy products, eggs, nuts and seeds, beans, and soy products.

The only problem with protein is that it tends to come wrapped up with a nutrient that is not so good for us—saturated fat. This kind of fat—found in beef, pork, and chicken, as well as in milk, cheese, and eggs—is the kind that promotes cardiovascular disease. Many of the eating tips you'll learn in this book are designed to help you develop the habit of getting more of your protein from sources that come with little or no saturated fat attached, such as fish, poultry breasts, nuts, and legumes.

Carbohydrates

Carbohydrates are fuel, plain and simple. Your body loves to burn carbohydrates and has an easy time doing so. In their simplest form, carbohydrates are sugar molecules. Sugar is pure carbohydrate. But so is a baked potato. Starch is just sugar in disguise. It is sugar molecules linked together into longer molecules. These longer molecules don't taste sweet on the tongue, but once they hit the stomach, they are quickly broken apart into sugar. (This is why when you roast vegetables or caramelize onions, they get sweeter; the cooking breaks down the starches into sugars.)

Now you understand the reason behind low-carb diets. All your life, you may have forced yourself, or your kids, to eat your rice and potatoes before you could have candy for dessert, when in reality they are the very same thing for your body.

But don't swear off bread quite yet. Your body loves carbohydrates. In fact, your energy comes from these sugar molecules being burned in each individual muscle cell. Like a little car engine, the "explosion" of the sugar molecule being burned is what makes your muscle cell expand and contract. For your muscles to work in any way, you need a steady supply of these sugar molecules.

However, your muscles can store only enough energy for about ninety seconds of exercise. Where does it come from after that? You don't have any built-in potato bins on your body.

The answer is fat.

Fat

For a long time, we thought fat made us fat. It only made sense. Fat in food must be easily stored in those handy fat deposits around your middle. And it's true; if your body gets more fat than it needs, it will store the rest. But it turns out the body is more clever than we suspected. If it gets extra protein or carbohydrates, it has no trouble converting those into fat storage, too. We now know that when it comes to weight gain, it doesn't matter in what form calories enter your body. Any excess calories get stored as fat.

Fat plays several roles in the body. It pads your organs and provides some insulation against cold, but its chief function is being your primary energy supply. When you exercise and use up the carbohydrates in your muscles in those first ninety seconds, your body turns to your fat stores for fuel. It liquidates the fat, breaks it back down into burnable molecules, and burns it for power. Yahoo! When we talk about burning fat during exercise, we mean it.

Many different types of fat exist in our food, but they can all be broken down into two categories: saturated and unsaturated. Saturated fat, which is solid at body temperature, is the bad guy. It clogs your arteries and leads to heart disease and strokes. Unsaturated fat, however—the kind that is liquid at body temperature—has a clean bill of health. It reduces cholesterol, keeps your heart healthy, and keeps you full. Most saturated fat comes from animals, and you know it when you see it: The marbling on your steak, as well as lard and butter, are saturated fat. Cooking oils are unsaturated fat.

You'll learn a lot more about fat during Week 3 of the program. For now, just keep in mind that a calorie of fat won't make you any fatter than a calorie of protein or carbs. It may, in fact, help you eat fewer calories overall.

THE PROBLEM WITH FAD DIETS

The people touting low-fat and low-carb diets know the truth about weight loss as well as anybody. They know that if calories in equal calories burned, weight stays the same, but if the amount of calories burned is higher, weight goes down. But they don't trust you to know what to do with the information. Instead, they try to give you a shortcut, one type of nutrient to focus on, and hope that by doing this, your other good eating habits will fall into place automatically.

The theories behind these two diet types are different. Low-fat diets are based on the fact that fat has more than twice as many calories per gram as do protein and carbohydrates. Fat is dense energy—which makes it a very convenient way for your body to store energy, but it also makes it a caloric powerhouse. Two tablespoons of butter or oil have more calories than a can of soda. Since fat is so dense with calories, dietitians have theorized that people can eat less fat and more carbohydrates, eat the same total weight of food, and consume fewer calories overall.

Unfortunately, these low-fat diets fail to take into account how people actually eat. The result has been an obesity disaster. When you replace fat with carbohydrates (which, remember, are really just sugars), the carbs are quickly absorbed into the blood, and blood-sugar levels spike. This leads to diabetes. It also leads to increased hunger, because your body becomes used to higher levels of blood sugar; whenever this drops, you feel hungry. Encouraging people to eat high proportions of carbohydrates has created a country of hummingbirds constantly craving more carbs to maintain their syrupy blood. As a result, we have become a nation of overeaters.

And then came Dr. Atkins. He was the first person to bring national attention to the damage caused by low-fat diets, and he showed that people could lose weight on his high-fat, low-carb diet. Because protein and fat are larger, more complex molecules than carbohydrates, the body takes a lot longer to digest them. A smaller amount of food will create a "slow burn" that doesn't spike blood-sugar levels and leaves you feeling full for a long time. Even though fat has more calories per gram than carbohydrates, Dr. Atkins believed that it would help people feel full on less and therefore they would eat fewer calories overall.

A lot of good has come from low-carb diets. But they have gone too far, by sending the message that people can eat as much fat and protein as they want as long as they stay away from carbs. Dr. Atkins thought that people's bodies would regulate appetite well if they weren't faced with spiking blood-sugar levels. He didn't count on how addicted to overeating we had already become. He underestimated our ability to pack away giant bunless cheeseburgers, or chef's salads soaking in blue cheese dressing. He didn't realize that a license to eat all the ham and butter you want might backfire.

And so here we are. We have learned important things from both the low-fat and low-carb diets, yet as a nation we are heavier than ever. Clearly, something is still missing from the weight-loss equation. And that something can't be packaged as a gimmick.

THE GOAL: BALANCE

I believe we have weathered the storm of fad diets and that a new era of nutritional common sense is dawning. We have the science we need and the wisdom of thirty years of dumb diets to guide us. We have come full circle on the diet merry-go-round, and we are coming back to some traditional notions of balance and moderation that might seem very familiar to our grandmothers.

As many people who tried low-carb diets have found, a lot of the fun of eating disappears along with the carbohydrates. Let's face it: A burger with the bun tastes a lot better than a burger without it. And you don't need to skip the bun! Just eat a smaller burger! And try veggies with that, not fries. Common sense. Traditional meals.

Nutritionists who push no-carb diets because they want you to avoid carb-induced spikes in blood-sugar levels don't consider that if some carbs are mixed in with protein and fat, they don't get digested instantly, because the body has to deal with the whole mix at once. That's right: Fat and protein can slow down the rate at which carbs are absorbed. As I said, no need to skip the bun!

One of the great advantages of eating a balanced diet is that it doesn't require so much attention on your part. I recommend a fairly equal balance between the three main nutrients, but don't get hung up on the numbers. You'll find that if you eat normally, in moderation, and stay away from pitfalls like junk food and dessert, this will take care of itself. Eat as people have done throughout time—a little meat, some grains, and lots of fruits and veggies—and don't worry about anything else. Don't count calories or carbs. No need to ask restaurants and sandwich shops for weird variations on what they normally serve.

Getting yourself back to a place where sensible eating comes naturally—undoing the programming done by fad diets, diet foods, and the allure of junk food—is what this program is all about. The best part of all may be that at the end of the six weeks it leaves you in a place where you need no help from anyone, and success comes automatically. Once you're cured, you're cured!

THE DIRTY DOZEN

Now that science has confirmed the health benefits of so many foods and the wisdom of eating a variety of natural ones, only a handful of foods are still on the wanted poster. For a simple and effective dieting guideline, just avoid these twelve food categories. You'd have to get creative to gain weight without these (which are all sources of either artery-clogging saturated fat or insulin-spiking refined carbohydrates).

Beef and Veal	Pork	Lamb
Bacon, Ham, and Sausage	Full-Fat Cheese	Butter and Margarine
White Flour	White Rice	Potatoes
Hydrogenated Vegetable Oil	Sugar	Sour Cream, Cream, and Whole-Fat Milk

4. Exercise: The Most Important Nutrient

Let's play a game. Read the following quote and see if you can guess who said it.

"We are underexercised as a nation. We look instead of play. We ride instead of walk. Our existence deprives us of the minimum of physical activity essential for healthy living."

Any guesses? I'll give you a hint: It was a president of the United States. Since it describes our current predicament so well, you might guess President Bush. Or maybe President Clinton. But you'd be way off. President John F. Kennedy uttered those words more than forty years ago. It may be shocking to hear that lack of exercise was considered a problem back then, because compared to us, that generation was a nation of superjocks.

If America was already turning into a country of couch potatoes in the early sixties, we have become almost indistinguishable from the couch today. Only one-third of adults gets the recommended bare minimum of a half hour of exercise each day. One-quarter of us gets no exercise at all.

Remember that energy-balance equation? So far, we've been focusing on the intake side—the amount of calories you eat. But the other side of the equation, the amount you burn, is equally important, if not more so. Those 335 extra calories a day we eat, compared with thirty years ago, are matched by an equivalent decline in the number we burn.

The culprits for this aren't just lack of planned exercises like walking, running, or biking. Much of our lack of exercise—and resulting obesity—can be chalked up to the many "conveniences" that now fill our lives. We never used to think of cooking a meal or raking leaves as exercise; they seemed too insignificant. But once enough of those insignificant activities are gone, we discover they added up to a significant calorie burn. Perhaps you order takeout, run the dishwasher, and use the time saved to get some walking in. Great, you burn the calories anyway. However, if you use the time these conveniences save to watch an extra hour of TV, you're in trouble.

In my videos, books, and on-line Walk Diets, I encourage people to get into a rhythm of walking two or three miles most days. I think this is the single most important "nutrient" you can add to your life—more so than unsaturated fat, whole-grain carbohydrates, or any multivitamin. In addition to this planned exercise, I'd love to see you develop the habit of rebelling against convenience. All those small activities your mother's generation did made a real difference. They help make a bridge connecting exercise and everyday life. Instead of making those things mutually exclusive concepts—we work a desk job to make money to buy time-saving gadgets that give us free time to exercise—use daily "chore" exercises to naturalize physical activity. They add up!

For example, simply cooking a homemade meal and then washing the dishes by hand burn about 130 more calories than do ordering takeout and using a dishwasher. It doesn't seem like a big deal when you're doing it, but over a year, you'll have saved thirteen pounds. You don't even need to be hard-core about it; do it most nights and save ten pounds a year. Of course, this is in addition to the huge benefits (in terms of health and lower-calorie meals) that come from eating home-cooked food. You'll hear about those throughout this book. But next time you're wavering about whether to cook dinner or not, don't forget to add your own calorie burn from cooking and cleanup into the equation.

WHAT'S SO GREAT ABOUT EXERCISE, ANYWAY?

Enough about numbers! I don't like to give them too much attention, because they can't possibly capture the complexity of life. Not everything can be expressed in a number, and that's especially true when it comes to exercise. The benefits of exercise go so far beyond calories burned that I almost don't know where to start.

Muscle seems like a good place. You've already heard how muscle is metabolically active (meaning it burns calories all the time), while fat isn't. The more fat you can convert to muscle, the more calories you will burn apart from your activities and exercise. While sitting, sleeping, and, yes, watching TV, your muscle continues at a low-grade burn. Get fit, and you'll burn two hundred additional calories per day through increased metabolism!

There is only one way on this planet to convert fat to muscle, and that is through good old-fashioned exercise. Your body is very good at adapting to your needs and giving you what you want. You signal to it what you want through behavior. When you use a muscle every day, your body starts building that muscle up so the task will be easier for you next time. Instead of converting the protein in your diet to fat and storing it for later, your body uses it to build the new muscle. Presto: less fat, more muscle.

Remember, your body likes to be thrifty with its calories. It won't burn them unless you give it a good reason to. (If you're exercising daily, your body assumes you need to for survival.) It would far prefer to hold on to as much fat as possible. Certain enzymes (molecular tools) are required to take apart your fat molecules and burn them as fuel, and the body isn't going to make these unless you give it a reason. This means that the more you exercise, the more the body gets used to burning fat. It makes more enzymes so that fat burning can start more quickly next time. This explains that profound unfairness we've all noticed: Fit people seem to burn off calories more easily than inactive people. It turns out they really do!

TONE IS EVERYTHING

When people learn that a half-hour walk will burn about two hundred calories, they sometimes think, Why bother? I can achieve the same thing by drinking one less bottle of Pepsi a day. Looking at the numbers, this is true, but it misses the bigger picture. Weight loss is not a goal in itself; it's a means to better health and better looks. Neither of those can be achieved by simply cutting way back on calories. We've all seen people who go on strenuous diets. Sure, they lose some weight, but they look sallow, their skin sags, and they have no muscle tone. (Their metabolisms will also slow down to adjust to their drastic change in caloric intake, stopping the weight loss but leaving them lethargic.) Forget the number on the scale; muscle tone is what makes people look good. Muscle holds its shape, while fat simply goes with gravity. I think we all know which we prefer!

Increasing muscle tone through exercise puts you in a wonderful feedback loop, where more exercise leads to more muscle and energy, which makes exercise come even easier, which builds more muscle, and on and on. The health benefits of exercise also vastly outweigh anything you get through simple dieting. Let's look at those now.

CARDIOVASCULAR DISEASE

Your blood vessels are just like the pipes in your house. Instead of carrying water, they carry blood. Normally, the walls of your blood vessels are nice and smooth so blood can flow through them unimpeded. In fact, your blood vessels can even expand to allow more blood to flow through them when necessary—a nice feature your house pipes don't yet have. Unfortunately, as your blood vessels get older, they lose some of this natural flexibility. And, like your house pipes, they also suffer from clogs. Grease buildup is a chief culprit with your sink drain, and it applies to your arteries, as well. Grease—which is saturated fat—solidifies, sticks to the lining of your blood vessels, and starts an obstruction that causes more fat and cholesterol molecules to stick as they go by. The obstruction grows and eventually can lead to a complete blockage of an artery. A blockage on the way to the heart causes a heart attack. A blockage on the way to the brain causes a stroke.

Exercise helps keep your cardiovascular system at peak health by working both your blood vessels and your heart. Making your blood vessels expand and contract regularly keeps them from hardening, so they can handle more blood flow with lower blood pressure. Exercise also makes your heart get stronger, and a stronger heart can handle a regular amount of blood flow with less effort. As if that wasn't enough, exercise improves your cholesterol profile, as well.

Cutting back on saturated fat in your diet, which we'll explore later in the book, is one of three great ways to reduce your risk of cardiovascular disease. The others are regular exercise and not smoking. Any one of these healthy actions cuts your risk of heart disease more or less in half. Obviously, the sane response is not to choose just one of these actions, but to do all three.

DIABETES

Diabetes is the most epidemic disease in America, with 60 million of us either diabetic or prediabetic. The causes are clear: lack of exercise and too much food, especially starches and sugars. When all those carbs hit the bloodstream, blood-sugar levels go sky-high. The pancreas starts producing insulin, which is the hormone "key" that opens up muscle cells so they can absorb sugar for energy. But they can take only so much, and after awhile they start to resist the action of the insulin. With blood-sugar levels rising, the pancreas pumps out even more insulin, desperately trying to force some cells to take the sugar. But insulin resistance keeps growing, too, and eventually the pancreas breaks down under the pressure. With little or no insulin being produced, blood-sugar levels rise catastrophically. Bam: You've got a case of full-blown diabetes.

High sugar levels in the blood wreak havoc on your blood vessels. The sugar hooks up with proteins in the blood, creating sticky molecules that attach to the sides of artery walls and form blockages. This explains why diabetics are at such high risk for heart attacks and strokes. In fact, two out of three diabetics will eventually die of heart disease. Sugary blood also causes particular damage to the kidneys, eyes, and brain.

Diabetes doesn't scare me, however, because I know it is one of the most treatable of conditions. The eating habits in this book will help you keep the flow of sugar into your blood slow and steady; the other half of the equation is to keep burning that sugar regularly through exercise. The more you use your muscles, the more muscles you develop, and the more sugar will be needed to fill them with energy. Regular use also primes your muscles to accept sugar more easily, so they can refuel quickly, which prevents insulin resistance from developing. Eat right, exercise regularly, and you can pretty much cross diabetes off your worry list.

BREAST CANCER

The link between exercise and cancer rate is small for most cancers, but breast cancer is an exception. Exercise at least four hours per week and your risk of breast cancer drops by a third! This is probably because exercise boosts your whole immune system and keeps your fat levels low. Exercise also helps prevent colon and prostate cancer.

OSTEOPOROSIS

One of the biggest fears women have as they age is of developing osteoporosis—weakening of the bones. Bones are made up of protein and calcium, and just as with muscle, exercise is the signal the body needs to put some resources into building up bone strength. If women don't exercise, after age thirty-five they start losing bone mass every year. By the time we reach our seventies, our bones can be severely brittle, meaning that simple falls result in breaks, breaks don't heal well, and our whole body slumps because the support structure just isn't there.

This happens only if you *don't* exercise. Keep exercising into your seventies and your bones will be as strong as those of women in their thirties. And, of course, get plenty of calcium in your diet (which almost all of us do anyway, and which you will certainly do if you develop the eating habits suggested in this book).

DEPRESSION AND STRESS

Tell me the last time you went for a walk, hike, or bike ride and felt really bad afterward. Tell me the last time you came home from exercising and said, "Gee, I'm really sorry I did that." It doesn't work that way. You *always* feel good after exercising. There's no better way to shake off stress and put yourself in better spirits. Studies show exercise to be every bit as good as drugs in relieving mild to moderate depression, with no side effects—unless you count weight loss! Then why don't doctors recommend it more? They do, but sadly, they have learned that too many people are more likely to take a pill than to walk a mile. Fortunately, you're not one of those people.

Why should exercise make us feel good? Because it causes feel-good chemicals like endorphins and anandamide to circulate through the brain, giving us a natural high. Also, stress causes a buildup of natural caffeinelike agitators in our bodies, and exercise gives us a way to burn off that steam naturally and get back to a relaxed state. Perhaps best of all, exercise usually gives us a brief escape from our regular thought patterns, letting us just be in our bodies for a while. All this adds up to the best mood fixer known. I recommend it daily!

OTHER CONDITIONS

Exercise is beneficial for whatever ails you. That's why women who walk regularly cut their risk of premature death from all causes in half! If there is a magic pill, this is it! Here are some more conditions that improve with exercise:

- **Immune System.** The cells of your immune system constantly circulate through your body, looking to eliminate invaders such as bacteria or cancer cells. Exercise boosts your number of immune cells and circulates them faster as your heart rate increases.
- **Alzheimer's Disease.** Older adults who walk more than two miles per day are only half as likely to develop Alzheimer's disease and other forms of dementia, compared with those who rarely walk. Why? Exercise regulates sugar levels in the brain, too, which prevents the formation of sticky substances that clog the brain's oxygen supply. Furthermore, we already know that exercise reduces stress, and scientists recently discovered that stress triggers enzymes in the brain that impair memory.
- **Arthritis.** Just as the wheel bearings on your car get rusty if they sit for too long, your joints need to be worked regularly through exercise. People with arthritis who keep exercising feel less pain and have more flexibility. Exercise can also reduce the inflammation caused by rheumatoid arthritis.
- **Digestive Diseases.** As with rheumatoid arthritis, digestive problems such as inflammatory bowel disease and Crohn's disease may be caused by an autoimmune response to inflammation, which can be alleviated by exercise.

A BEGINNER'S GUIDE TO WALKING

Now that you know how wonderful walking is for you, you'll want to make it a regular part of your life. Walking has always been my exercise of choice for several reasons:

- Everybody knows how to do it. In fact, you've been practicing for years!
- The health benefits of exercises more strenuous than walking are minor.
- Walking is something you can keep doing your entire life.

THE EXERCISE SCORECARD
Walk regularly and you can count on the following benefits.

Metabolism (calories burned): ↑ 200 calories every day—not including your exercise!

Risk of heart disease: ↓ 45%

Risk of stroke: ↓ 42%

Risk of diabetes: ↓ 58%

Risk of Alzheimer's: ↓ 42%

Risk of premature death: ↓ 55%

Many people who buy this book will have already been walking for years, either with my books and videos or on their own program. If you are one of those people, keep doing what you've been doing! You already know what a huge improvement it's made in your life.

If you haven't been on a regular walking program, start immediately! Trying to lose weight and get fit by changing your eating habits but not exercising would be like trying to walk with one leg tied up. To learn everything you need to know about walking, and to begin a program that will start you off gently and help you gradually build endurance, the best place to go is my first book, *Walk Away the Pounds*. In addition to the basic program, you'll learn about safety issues and health conditions, motivation techniques, the benefits of simple strength training, and much more.

For people who want to get started right away, the following guide should be enough to get you up and walking in no time. Enjoy!

THE BENEFITS OF INDOOR WALKING

Nothing is more invigorating than a brisk walk in crisp fall air, and I think you should seize the opportunity to take one any chance you get. Still, I find that most people do best if they spend most of their exercise time on indoor walking, for the following reasons:

- There are no excuses for skipping the walk, such as rain or heat.
- You can multitask, watching TV while walking, or sneaking it in while your toddler naps.

- Walking in place allows you to employ a variety of side and back steps that work a broader range of muscles than forward walking.
- You can exercise in complete privacy.

SAFETY AND HEALTH CONCERNS

Walking is incredibly safe. Our bodies were designed to walk; the stress on our joints and muscles is mild, so injuries are rare. This isn't true for exercises like running, biking, or aerobics, where foot and leg injuries are surprisingly common. The gentle nature of walking also makes it ideal for people with health concerns who need to start exercising without aggravating their conditions. Hardly a condition exists that isn't *improved* by walking. Of course, if you have health questions of any kind, you should check with your physician before beginning any exercise program. Here's the scoop on a few common conditions and what you might need to consider.

Heart Disease

Moderate walking puts no dangerous stress on your heart. In fact, it's one of the best ways to improve your cholesterol, blood pressure, and heart strength. If you have a heart condition, talk to your physician about beginning a walking program right away.

High Blood Pressure or Cholesterol

As with heart disease, walking is the best way to improve cardiovascular conditions without risk.

Diabetes

Walking is a terrific way to burn blood sugar and thus reduce or eliminate your need for insulin shots. However, exercise can trigger a rise in blood-sugar levels at first, as your body starts transforming its fat into sugar and sending it through your blood to your muscles for energy. If your diabetes is advanced, you may need to take a shot of insulin before exercising. You should also drink water beforehand. Ask your doctor what will be best for your situation.

Arthritis

If you are having a particularly painful flare-up in any joints that will be impacted by walking, it's a good idea to lay off the exercise for the time being. Once you're better, walking can help keep your joints loose and less painful.

Dizziness or Fainting

If you suffer from regular dizziness or fainting, you and your doctor should determine the cause before you begin any exercise program.

GEAR

Another plus of walking—especially indoor walking—is that you need no special equipment. A decent pair of sneakers, your rattiest shorts and T-shirt, and away you go. Still, there are some pointers on gear you may find helpful.

Shoes

Don't try to walk in cheap shoes. Every mile you walk is 2,000 steps; it only makes sense to give your feet good support for all that impact. If you are uncomfortable or get blisters, you're more likely to stop walking. A small investment in good sneakers is the most affordable health insurance you'll ever find.

Look for shoes that are tight against your instep but leave wiggle room for your toes, that cushion your heel and pad, and that have an arch that matches your foot's natural architecture. Even good shoes start to break down after a year of heavy use, so replace yours when necessary.

Socks

Good socks can make more difference than you think. New cotton socks are usually fine, but as they get older, they compress (meaning less cushioning) and stretch out (meaning they'll bunch up and give you blisters). Cotton also traps more moisture than modern synthetics that are designed to wick away moisture. And moisture leads to blisters. If you suffer from blisters or sweaty feet when you walk, try out a set of wick-away socks.

Pedometer

There are three ways to measure your walking. You can measure distance (easiest if you walk outside or use my videos), time, or steps. Steps are the easiest of all to measure. A pedometer is a device that clips to your sneaker or belt and counts every step you take during the day. Knowing that 2,000 steps is a mile, you would walk two miles by going until your pedometer reads 4,000. You can also track your total steps during the day for all activities, and set your goal that way. An excellent goal for weight loss is 10,000 total steps a day, though that's not easy to achieve without structured walking. Pedometers are available at discount or sporting-goods stores, or through www.LeslieSansone.com.

Hand Weights, Ab Belts, and Stretch Bands

Walking does a great job of toning your lower half and giving you super cardiovascular and mood-lifting benefits, but it doesn't do much for your upper half. That's why I recommend some gentle strength training while you walk. Two-pound hand weights, ab belts with handles and rubber cords that you stretch while you walk, and versatile rubber stretch bands are three ways to achieve this. You can use them all for variety or pick whichever feels most comfortable. For information on each, as well as the special benefits of strength training, see my book *Walk Away the Pounds* or my Web site (www.lesliesansone.com).

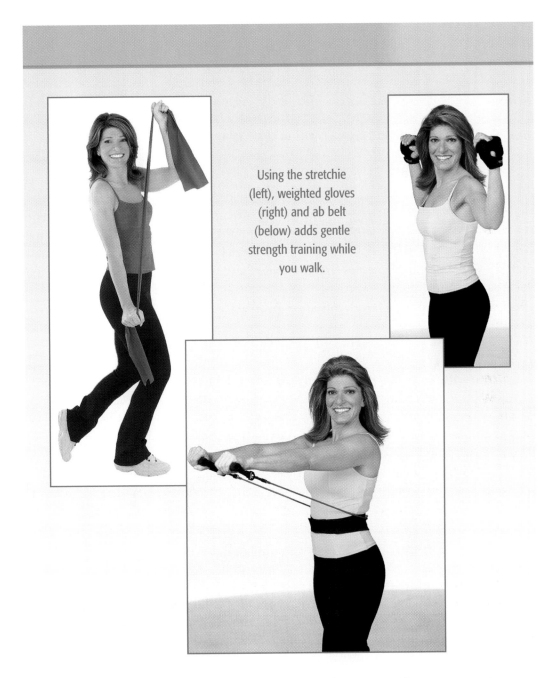

Using the stretchie (left), weighted gloves (right) and ab belt (below) adds gentle strength training while you walk.

Basic Walking Moves

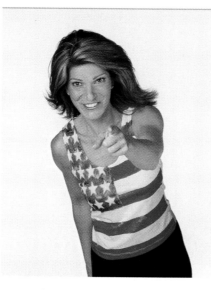

There are four basic steps that I work into all my walks. Mixing these steps into your routine ensures that you engage as many muscles as possible. It also keeps you energized! The first step is about as basic as it gets.

WALK IN PLACE

Begin each workout by walking as you normally do. You know how to walk, but you can check my form for pointers. My foot is raised perhaps six inches off the ground, and my opposite arm swings forward at the same time. It's essential to have good upright posture while walking—or doing anything else, for that matter! Your abdominal muscles should be tight and your shoulder blades retracted to get that beautiful spinal alignment that prevents sore backs. One thing you'll find about walking in place is that you end up lifting your knees higher than if you're walking forward.

Choose your pace based on your abilities and goals. However long or fast you intend to go, begin each walk with several minutes of gentle warm-up. This is vitally important in order to get your blood pumping through your muscles and fluid lubricating your joints. Warming up not only prevents injuries but also allows your muscles to perform at a higher level without tiring, so it will make you a better, stronger walker.

Once you feel your heart starting to pick up, increase your pace. Pump your arms to get your upper body involved and to boost the calorie burn. (This also helps your balance.) The right pace for you is whatever keeps you in that middle rate of exertion, where you can pass the "talk test"—you aren't gasping, can talk if necessary, but your lungs are working harder than normal. I usually

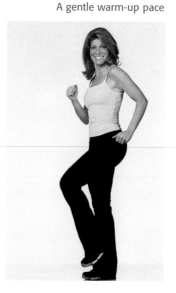

A gentle warm-up pace

try to get people walking at about two steps per second, which works out to about a fifteen-minute mile. That's pretty fast! It may be too brisk for you at first, but you'll work up to it in no time.

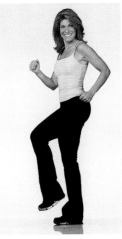

A good midwalk pace, with the foot nice and high for extra calorie burn

SIDE STEPS

After a few minutes of walking in place, you are ready to mix in some side steps. These are a great way to work your thighs and backside to get that nicely sculpted core. The pace is ever so slightly slower than walking in place, because the motion takes longer.

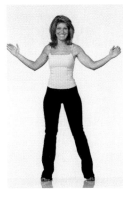
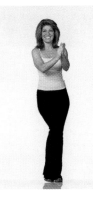
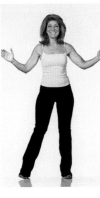
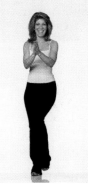

1. STEP TO YOUR LEFT with your left foot, continuing to face forward. Your arm action should mirror your legs: Spread them wide as you step.

2. BRING YOUR RIGHT foot together with your left. Bring your hands together at the same time.

3. STEP BACK TO YOUR RIGHT with your right foot, spreading your arms again.

4. BRING YOUR LEFT FOOT together with your right foot. Bring your hands together at the same time.

Repeat this four-step move ten times; then return to walking in place for another minute or two; then do another ten side steps. Now you are beginning to see why walking in place allows you to do things you could never do on an outdoor walk! Once you are comfortable with these two basic steps, you are ready to work the third step into your routine.

KICKS

Kicks give the quadriceps (the front thigh muscles) and backside a little extra workout. The four-step move is similar to that for side steps.

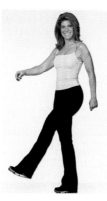 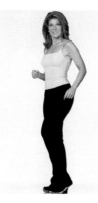 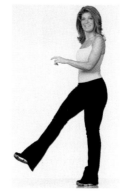 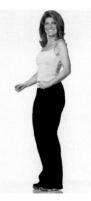

1. KICK YOUR LEFT LEG forward at a comfortable distance.

2. BRING YOUR FOOT BACK to the ground.

3. KICK YOUR RIGHT LEG forward at a comfortable distance.

4. BRING YOUR FOOT BACK to the ground.

The kick shouldn't break you out of your pace. You aren't trying to pull a Bruce Lee move on anybody. Also make sure you don't lean back when kicking; if you lean back, you won't get the full muscle benefit. Repeat this four-step move ten times; then return to walking in place. Continue to mix in one or two minutes of walking in place with ten counts of side steps and kicks (always returning to walking in place in between). Once you are comfortable with these three basic steps, you are ready to work the fourth step into your routine.

KNEE LIFTS

The knee lift gives you the benefits of walking and crunches at the same time. Bringing your legs up with every step really works the abs and quads. The four-step motion is identical to that of the kicks, except you lift your knee up instead of kicking your foot out.

Repeat this four-step move ten times; then return to walking in place. You now have the four basic moves down and should mix them all into your routines.

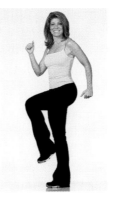

1. LIFT YOUR LEFT KNEE until it is nearly horizontal.

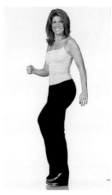

2. BRING IT BACK DOWN.

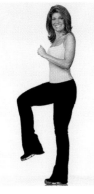

3. LIFT YOUR RIGHT KNEE until it is nearly horizontal.

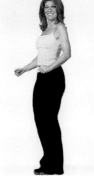

4. BRING IT BACK DOWN.

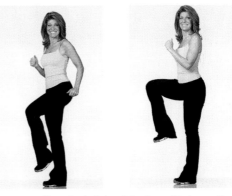

You can adjust the height of the knee lift depending on your abilities. Note the less strenuous lift in the first picture and then the perfectly horizontal lift in the second—yeah, girl!

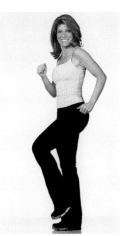

A nice relaxed cool-down stride

COOL DOWN

An essential part of healthy walking is the cool-down period at the end. During the last few minutes of your walk, reduce your intensity until you are back to that gentle warm-up pace. This allows you to bring your heartbeat back to its regular rate in a gradual fashion, preventing the situation where your muscles have stopped working but your heart is still pounding in your chest.

The Flex Questionaire

You are unique, and so is the solution to your weight-loss issues. The Flex Questionnaire is your way of identifying where your issues lie so that you can tweak the six-week program to make it suit your needs. It's easy. Just read each of the statements below and do the following:

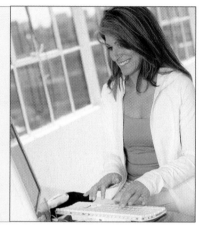

If you agree strongly with the statement, write a **2** in the blank.

If you agree somewhat with the statement, write a **1** in the blank.

If you disagree with the statement, write a **0** in the blank.

Then look below to interpret your results.

_____ 1. I use the clock to decide when to eat.

_____ 2. I frequently skip breakfast or just have a bagel or piece of toast.

_____ 3. I often feel stuffed after dinner.

_____ 4. My dinner often comes from a restaurant or take-out place, or is out of a box.

_____ 5. Part of my weight-loss strategy involves skipping meals.

_____ 6. When I eat out, I try to get the most for my money.

_____ 7. I'd exercise more if I didn't find it so boring.

_____ 8. Sometimes I eat because I'm bored, sad, anxious, or stressed.

_____ 9. I feel hungry or have low concentration at midmorning.

_____ 10. I often take seconds at a meal.

_____ 11. I rarely have time to cook a meal from scratch.

_____ 12. I keep junk food in my house, glove compartment, or desk drawer.

_____ 13. I like restaurants with Atkins-friendly menus, because then I don't have to worry about what I order.

_____ 14. I'd rather lose weight by eating less than by burning more calories.

_____ 15. When I get offered food (such as at a party), I take it, even if I'm not hungry.

_____ 16. I need several cups of caffeine to get through the day.

____ 17. As long as I stay away from carbs, I can eat whatever I want.

____ 18. I eat my vegetables because they're good for me, but I don't really enjoy them.

____ 19. A meal feels incomplete if it doesn't include dessert.

____ 20. When I eat out, I want to indulge myself.

____ 21. I don't like exercising, because it leaves me sweaty and exhausted.

____ 22. I eat my meals while watching TV or working.

____ 23. I rarely eat brown rice, whole wheat, or other whole grains.

____ 24. I usually clear my plate.

____ 25. Vegetables are too time-consuming to prepare.

____ 26. I regularly eat in bed, in the car, or at my desk.

____ 27. It's rude to split entrées or order a small amount of food at a restaurant.

____ 28. My day is simply too packed to squeeze any exercise in.

____ 29. I don't like to waste food, even unhealthy food.

____ 30. I don't eat many eggs, because they are bad for me.

____ 31. I stay away from olive oil, other vegetable oils, and nuts, because they are too fattening.

____ 32. I eat my meal in fifteen minutes or less.

____ 33. Sometimes I get so hungry waiting for my next meal that I'll devour anything within reach.

____ 34. I would eat more fish if I knew more interesting ways to cook it.

____ 35. I'm too out of shape to begin exercising now.

TABULATING YOUR SCORE

Fill in your answers in the table below, then add up each column, and write your scores on the next page. Each category is the focus of one week in the six-week program (except exercise, which is an ongoing focus).

A	B	C	D	E	F	G
1. ___	2. ___	3. ___	4. ___	5. ___	6. ___	7. ___
8. ___	9. ___	10. ___	11. ___	12. ___	13. ___	14. ___
15. ___	16. ___	17. ___	18. ___	19. ___	20. ___	21. ___
22. ___	23. ___	24. ___	25. ___	26. ___	27. ___	28. ___
29. ___	30. ___	31. ___	32. ___	33. ___	34. ___	35. ___

Column A:	Intentional Eating Habit	_____
Column B:	Breakfast Habit	_____
Column C:	Portion-Control Habit	_____
Column D:	Slow-Food Habit	_____
Column E:	Snack Habit	_____
Column F:	Restaurant Habit	_____
Column G:	Exercise Habit	_____

INTERPRETING YOUR RESULTS

The higher the number in each category, the more you need to pay attention to that aspect of behavior (or to the category of healthy food featured in the chapter for that behavior). Here's a general guideline:

0–2   You have this area under control. Good for you!

3–5   This is an issue for you. Things aren't disastrous yet, but you could definitely improve your health and waistline with some attention to this area.

6–7   You have a problem in this area. Pay special attention to the chapter dealing with it, and make an extra effort to adopt as many of the behavior strategies as possible.

8–10   You are in crisis. You can't go on this way. Start the program with the chapter covering this topic and keep working on this area for as many weeks as it takes to get it under control before moving on to the other chapters.

TAKING ACTION

Having identified the areas you need to focus on, you are ready to begin the six-week program. Having a sense of where your issues lie will help you decide how intensely to focus on each lifestyle change. Each week includes six different behavior suggestions that can help you develop a smart eating habit. I hope you'll try them all, but I certainly don't expect you to adopt them all. For instance, if this questionnaire has helped you determine that you already have healthy breakfast habits but that portion control is a major issue for you, then you might fly through Week 2 (breakfast), playing around with a couple of my breakfast suggestions but not changing what already works for you; then, when you get to Week 3 (portion control), you'll want to make a concerted effort to try all my suggestions and really change your patterns. You might even spend some of Week 2 getting a head start on portion control. By flexing the plan, you can make sure that it pays the biggest dividends where you need them most.

THE HONESTY PAGE

Tests in which people assess themselves are notoriously unreliable. It's easy to see where the questions are leading and to change your answers to make yourself happier. So here's an extra question to help you decide if you have any "hidden" problem areas. List your meals and exercise over the past seven days on the next page. You won't be able to remember every one, but do the best you can. Don't worry about which particular day you ate something; no one's memory is that good. And don't forget to include snacks, desserts, and drinks.

Now, *don't* protest that last week was unusual. Every week is unusual in one way or another. (And remember, this is just between you and the page.) If you did something last week, chances are you'll do it again. What patterns can you see in your week? Are you skipping breakfast? Avoiding exercise? Snacking incessantly? This is your chance to be incredibly honest with yourself and to say, Yeah, I see a problem in my eating behaviors last week. Then add that to the special areas of concern you identified in the questionnaire, even if it didn't seem like a problem from the way you answered it.

GET STARTED!

You've spent the past several chapters learning a little about nutrition, exercise, and yourself. Supported by all that knowledge, you are ready to dig into six weeks that will change your life. No holding back. Get ready. Get set. Get started!

The Honesty Page

Breakfasts	Lunches	Dinners	Snacks and Desserts	Drinks	Exercise

PART II

SIX WEEKS TO
A NEW YOU

6. How to Use the Six-Week Food Plan

I don't have any idea what your favorite foods are. I don't have a clue how early you wake up, how big a breakfast you eat, or how loudly the Almond Joy bars sing to you from the candy cliffs of the checkout line. So how can I possibly design an ideal food plan for *you*?

The answer is that I can't. But you can. And over the next six weeks, you will. My job is to give you the tools, tips, and information you need to develop automatic eating and exercise habits that let you lose weight, get healthy, and stay energized without taking up too much of your mental real estate. You might think of it as the "mindless" diet, because once it's up and running, you shouldn't have to give it much thought at all!

Each week, I'll introduce you to one of the six habits that keep people naturally slender. I'll explain how each habit works and why they are all win-win situations: big impact on your waistline, minimal inconvenience in your day.

Each week, I also focus on one type of food that can make a big difference in your goals. Not only do these foods provide fantastic nutrition; they also help you eat less but feel full longer. They give you more energy, improved metabolism, better health, and a whole different body.

Then it is up to you. Each day of the week, you get a Day Page; it's the easiest

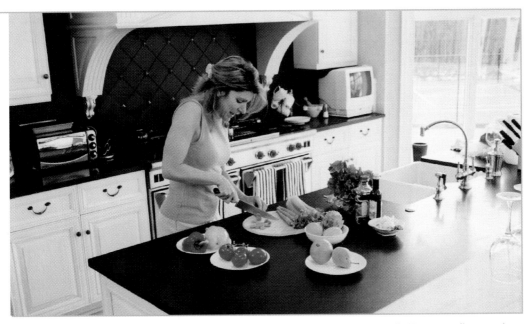

Food is your friend! Especially if you eat all your colors.

way to keep yourself on task and to track your progress. Each Day Page includes the following sections:

MISSION

Whatever the habit you're working on that week, each day I suggest one simple way of putting it into practice. For example, if the focus is smart restaurant habits, I might ask you to go out to dinner with a friend and split one entrée and one dessert—no exceptions. Or I might have you go to a fast-food restaurant for lunch and order the healthiest item on the menu, the thing you would never even consider. Whatever the suggestion, you're not required to make it a regular part of your life yet. Just give it a try; then go back to the Day Page and mark the box to show that you completed your mission for that day.

WALK BOX

If you know me, you know I'm all about exercise. This isn't because I'm some kind of marathoner hooked on the "runner's high"; it's because I'm constantly amazed how something so simple and pleasurable as a daily walk can have such an incredible impact on my shape, health, and attitude. It wouldn't be a Leslie Sansone plan if it didn't include a daily walk, and this is your place to record how far you went and how it felt.

FOOD FOCUS

Just as the way to develop smart habits is to work them into your life gradually, the way to work healthy foods into your eating routines is to try them out. Each day, I suggest a couple of easy recipes featuring that week's food focus. The recipes are simple and delicious, because the goal is to be able to show your family (or yourself) how these foods can add fun and excitement to your diet. For example, if the food focus for the week is good fat, I might suggest the Tuna and Radish Salad with Creamy Avocado Dressing. Once you've tasted it, you may never go back to your old salads!

You get to choose between two recipes each day—or substitute another using that same food. Life is complicated, so I want you to have as much flexibility as possible when figuring out the best way to incorporate the food into your day. You'll know what works for you.

NUTRITION CENTER

The Nutrition Center gives you space to record everything you eat during the day. And I mean *everything*. This is no time for creative memory lapses; you'll only be cheating yourself. Besides, you don't need to count calories or do anything else official with this record. I've never found that kind of pressure helpful, and I firmly believe that you're responsible enough to look at the facts and know what needs to be done. The challenge is getting the facts down—we all slip up if we wait too long to record what we ate. Oh yeah, you think, there was that bag of pretzels before lunch. . . . And yes, I did buy that brownie at the school bake sale. . . . I don't think I ate or drank anything while watching TV last night . . . or did I? Consider carrying this book with you throughout the day so that you can record what you eat while it's fresh in your mind. If you don't think you have a problem remembering, you can take a few minutes at the end of the day to record your food intake.

And don't forget your water intake. Those eight little glass icons at the bottom of the Nutrition Center aren't for tracking eggnog! Make sure you cross one out every time you drink a glass of water, and aim to have all eight crossed out by the end of the day. That means spacing your water intake out through the day, because drinking six glasses of water right before bed is a bad idea!

NOTES

Because life is about more than food, and because everything in life is connected, I wanted to make sure you had some space each day to write anything that came to mind. This is your free space to record your hopes and dreams—or just to remind yourself to take out the trash! You might want to use the Notes section to jot down circumstances that affected your ability to accomplish your eating and exercise goals. For instance, you might write, "Tried a morning walk today and went three miles for the first time! Had great energy! Maybe try walking in morning more often?" Or: "Huge plate of pasta for lunch made me sleepy all afternoon. Drank too much coffee to stay alert. Try chicken salad for lunch tomorrow." *Writing down* what's going on in your head, and in your life, makes it so much more concrete, which makes it much easier to deal with. Use the Notes as your tool for staying in touch with yourself.

SUNDAY WRAP-UP

This is *your* plan. That's why it's so important to customize the plan to fit your lifestyle and your goals. Maybe your goal is simply to lose ten pounds and reduce your risk of diabetes and cardiovascular disease by cutting down on refined carbs and saturated fat. In that case, you should feel free to ignore certain parts of the plan and accentuate others.

I don't expect you to adopt every habit in this book or to embrace every new food. That really would monopolize your life! No, the point of trying out six different tricks each week is so you can find two or three that make a big difference. Those are the ones to take with you into the following week, and the PERFECT Support System will help you do that.

Every Sunday, instead of exercising, tracking your nutrition, and working on your habits, your only task is to use the PERFECT Support System to determine what worked for you that week, what didn't, and what might have worked if it had been done a little differently. Eat anything you want. Lounge by the pool all day. Just be sure to crack open this book to the Sunday Wrap-Up to take stock of your progress, set your goals for the upcoming week, and reinforce your new habits with celebration, gratitude, and reminders of how you've changed already.

Think you can do that? Of course you can! Not only is it easy; it's fun, too. And that might be the most important trick to making a new habit stick. You'll find that with no pressure applied, and no penalty for setbacks, your successes build effortlessly. So what are you waiting for? Week 1 lies just around the bend!

HEALTH FLASH

The spicier or more strongly flavored a food is, the less you tend to eat—though you still feel just as full afterward. Possibly your body needs only so much total "flavor" before it feels full. Or maybe the strong spice makes you eat more slowly, so you feel full before you've had a chance to stuff yourself. Either way, this is a great reason to have a heavy hand with the salsa, garlic, or curry.

7. Week 1
The Intentional Eating Habit

On your mark! Get set! Take a deep breath . . . and say grace.

That's right, the very first step on your road to sensible eating and weight loss is simply to say grace before your next meal.

Before you fling this book out the window, let me explain. Saying grace can be done in a hundred different ways. Whether it's a traditional grace or a moment of silence before you begin eating, it involves reeling your mind in from wherever it's been wandering and making it present at the table, so eating becomes a conscious act.

I call this *intentional eating,* and it's the opposite of the kind of eating we so often do while driving, working, or watching TV: hand to bag to mouth, hand to bag to mouth. No brain required. This mindless eating is one of the major culprits in America's obesity problem. If we ate only when we were really and truly hungry, and stopped eating when we were full, weight control would not be a problem.

The challenge comes because there

are so many reasons other than hunger that cause us to eat. You know them. Emotional eating is a biggie. At some point in life, often in childhood, many of us learned that eating can temporarily distract us from sadness or anxiety—even though it ultimately leads to more unhappiness when it causes weight gain. Others experience the flip side of emotional eating, especially those who experienced real, prolonged hunger at some point in their lives. They don't eat because food feels good, but because they've learned to fear that first rumble in their tummy.

Other types of mindless eating may seem minor compared to the intense issues of emotional eating, but they can pile on just as many calories when the day is done. If you feel that you have to eat during certain activities, or have to clear your plate, or have to eat when the clock strikes a certain number, then you are eating mindlessly. Becoming aware of when you do it, and learning to take control of those habits, can be the key to permanent weight loss.

What we're really talking about is changing the nature of the power relationship between you and your food. You may have grown accustomed to the judgment—whether self-imposed or first delivered by a family member—that you have no control when it comes to food. Once you believe this, of course you're going to keep eating half a gallon of ice cream. Why fight it? After all, you have no control.

In truth, you have perfect control over what you put in your mouth. The problem comes when you allow your brain to check out; then the eating autopilot kicks in. If you can stay present and continue to be aware of your feelings as you eat, then you are much less likely to surrender to food. People who, halfway through a meal, are asking themselves, Does this taste good? Am I still enjoying it? How much more do I want? are the ones who stay slim for life.

Breaking your patterns of automatic eating is going to make you enjoy food more, because you'll become aware of sensations and flavors you've been taking for granted. It's like when you go away on vacation and then come back and find that familiar things feel so good again.

Eating intentionally does not mean forgoing dessert or not clearing your plate of delicious food; it just means being aware of why you do it. Let the impulse to eat come from you, not the chocolate cake in the kitchen.

SIX STRATEGIES FOR DEVELOPING YOUR INTENTIONAL EATING HABIT

1. SAY GRACE

Saying grace before a meal—almost every culture has its own version of doing this—helps remind you of all the important things in life. How miraculous it is that you and your family are lucky enough to be alive on this Earth, sustained by the bounty of nature. Reminding yourself of how you, your food, your community (who produced the food), the natural world, and the source of creation are all connected can go a long way toward changing the dynamics of your relationship to food. Whatever way you do it, it's simply a great habit, one that will add depth and meaning to all your eating experiences.

Saying grace doesn't need to be a big deal. It can be a private moment of silent reflection for you, or a shared ritual for everyone at the table. Either way, not only will it make eating a more spiritual experience; it will also make you enjoy your food more. It sets the mood for a level of mindfulness you can maintain throughout the meal. Chew your food. *Taste* your food. Give blessings all around you.

2. Get Hungry

There have been times when cheesecake looked downright repulsive to me. Those times were usually after I'd just eaten a piece—or two. And there have been times when I was so famished that a bag of pretzels from the vending machine was like a revelation. What's the number-one secret to making your food more delicious? Be hungry when you eat it!

With food being ever present in most of our lives, we tend to get used to that comforting feeling of fullness all the time. Correspondingly, any sensation of hunger makes us panic: Low blood sugar! Shaking hands! Irritability! Must eat now! Learning to get over this fear is an important step in mastering self-control.

As with other bodily sensations—like being cold, hot, or sleepy—hunger is just a message from your body to your brain, an update. It isn't an order. You are in charge. What you do with the information is entirely up to you.

So often we eat because "it's eating time," or because we see food and respond automatically. By learning to recognize your body's hunger signals, and to put them in their place, you'll realize how often you eat when you're not really hungry. That will start to seem mighty strange to you. Eventually, you'll stop! Your body will say, Yes, everyone else in the office is having a piece of birthday cake, but I'm not hungry, so why eat now? As you know, there will be plenty of other birthday cakes in the office; someday you may be hungry for one. Wait for that one; it'll taste best.

3. Food Is Not Love

Bless our mothers. So many of them cooked great meals as one of their many ways of nurturing us. It's only natural that we'd come to associate food with those feelings of safety, comfort, and love. That can be a great thing. Food and meals have an important place in the family. But sometimes as adults, we can look to food as a substitute for love. If we're going through a bad stretch, and crave the simplicity and comfort of childhood, food can be a quick fix, especially foods we ate as children. Nothing wrong with that. Only when food becomes an ongoing emotional crutch does it lead to eating bouts and weight gain.

If you find that your bouts of overeating happen when you're sad or lonely, then you know that food is an emotional trigger for you. Before you can develop your intentional eating habit, you need to separate food from love. Making food an unemotional issue will make it much easier to deal with.

Many people have found success in controlling their eating by discovering a much more powerful source of love within them—love from a higher power. This is the approach of Overeaters Anonymous, an organization that follows the same twelve-step program as Alcoholics Anonymous. Recognizing that the power to overcome an overeating habit can come from divine support, instead of from your own willpower, helps remove the guilt and self-blame. And once the psychological edge is removed, food can go back to being just food. Then you can put it in its place—a much smaller place in your life.

4. Food Is Not Background Music

If you are truly present whenever you eat, it becomes impossible to treat food as so many of us do—as an accompaniment to the rest of our lives. Endlessly munching popcorn as we watch TV, or M&Ms while we drive, or chips while we work, is the worst kind of automatic behavior, because you are consuming loads of calories and *you're not even really enjoying it*. You don't need a constant trickle of food and drink to get through the day. If boredom is the problem, boredom plus junk food is not the solution. As you track your food intake in your Day Pages, you'll get a sense of whether "invisible" calories are contributing unwanted pounds.

5. If It Doesn't Taste Good, Don't Eat It

How often do you eat things you aren't excited about? Why do you? Because you feel like you are doing something wrong if you don't clear your plate? Do you stuff down a "balanced dinner" so that you can treat yourself to dessert as a reward? If so, it might actually be better to eat just dessert for dinner (assuming you can get enough vitamins and nutrients in your other meals). Now there's a revolutionary idea!

Try to deprogram all automatic patterns you bring to the table. Do you throw some chips or potato salad next to your sandwich for lunch because the sandwich looks too plain by itself? Because you always have to have a side dish? Do you eat the bun with your burger when all you really want is the burger? Getting in touch with exactly what your body wants, and letting that be in charge, rather than social customs, is one of the best ways to remind yourself exactly who is in power here.

Turning off the assembly line is another important intentional eating behavior. You know the assembly-line mentality: As soon as a forkful of food goes in the mouth, the fork is back at the plate, digging out the next bite so it'll be ready to shovel in as soon as you swallow. We all do this, but it's a habit that can be broken. Next time you eat, try this: Take a bite of food; then put your fork down on your plate. Chew your food slowly; enjoy the taste. Only once you have swallowed can you pick up your fork to work on bite number two. This also applies to finger food: Eat one nut at a time, be aware of how good it tastes, and don't pick up another until the first one is gone. No one's racing.

6. Eat for the Future

A big part of growing up is learning to do things because of how they make us feel later. Staying up until the wee hours of the morn may be fun when we're twenty, but once we're a little older, we realize that the price we pay the next day isn't worth it. Children can't resist the instant gratification of an ice-cream cone, but we know they need to get some real food in them first or they'll crash later on.

Unfortunately, when it comes to our own eating, we have more trouble learning this lesson. Our stomachs seem to be hard-wired for instant gratification. Training your body to desire foods that provide long-lasting fulfillment, rather than the short-lived pleasure of French onion dip, is perhaps the most important step in developing naturally slimming eating habits, but it doesn't happen automatically. After all, rare is the person who looks up from her desk at noon and thinks, I feel an overwhelming urge for a plate of spinach!

Yet we all know food isn't just about the sensation it gives you the instant it hits your tongue; it's about keeping you satisfied, energized, and on an even keel all day long. Just as a case of food poisoning from egg salad can put you off hard-boiled eggs for months, your body learns to connect foods with how they make you feel later on—if it's paying attention. You'll stop craving the fast food at lunch when you start automatically associating it with the grease-laden, carb-heavy slump you feel in the afternoon. And you'll truly start to crave the spinach salad. You might not be conscious of why, and it hardly matters; you'll just be trusting your body's innate wisdom.

Water

I have a magic potion. It's crystal clear and beautiful. When you swirl it, it catches the light and sparkles, giving a hint of the powerful life fluid within. I use it for many wonderful purposes—and so do you. What you might not be using it for, however, is weight loss. In many ways, it's the foundation of health and fitness, which is why it's our first dietary focus. You have no excuse for not trying it out; it's widely available and amazingly cheap, even free—right out of your tap!

The magic potion is water, of course, and we need about eight glasses a day. We generally get that much, too. The problem is that we rarely get it straight up. Instead, it comes muddied in a mix of sugar syrup or alcohol, both of which are chock-full of calories.

The average American consumes about 450 calories per day in drinks. Sodas lead the list at 200 calories per day, followed by alcohol and milk at 100 each and juice at 50. Since we know that 10 calories per day equals 1 pound of body weight per year, cutting 450 drink calories from your daily diet would mean losing 45 pounds per year—without altering your meals at all! (This assumes that your weight has been stable. If you are still consuming more calories than you burn, the 45 pounds would first apply to stopping that weight gain.)

If you are going to use my magic potion to eliminate just one type of drink, make it sodas. While milk, juice, and alcohol in moderation all contribute to health, soda has no redeeming value whatsoever. It delivers floods of sugar into your bloodstream, causing insulin levels to surge, and then gets converted into fat. With thirty grams or more of sugar per serving, soda is the fast track to diabetes. But the nasty impact of soda goes even further. Soda is full of phosphoric acid, which must be buffered in the digestive tract. Calcium is the best way to do this. Where does your body get that calcium? From your bones. A steady diet of soda leaches calcium from your bones, contributing to osteoporosis.

If you are a soda drinker, figure out how many bottles a day you drink; then add up the calories and divide by ten. The number you get is how many pounds a year you can lose merely by switching to the magic potion.

Water encourages healthy weight in many other indirect ways, as well. This only makes sense, since women's bodies are 60 percent water. Drinking enough water allows us to keep that percentage nice and high. If we don't drink enough and therefore become dehydrated, fatigue is one of the first symptoms to hit, because water is responsible for ferrying nutrients to our muscles and brain. And when we feel fatigued, we sometimes think we are low on energy and need a snack. We don't. The energy is there; it just isn't getting to your cells. Fill up with water and everything starts running normally again. You've revived yourself without consuming a calorie!

Water also helps expand our stomachs and makes us feel full, again without consuming a calorie. Water is a smart way to fill your stomach during meals so that you eat smaller portions. True, the water disappears from your stomach fairly quickly, but by then your body is receiving plenty of "full" signals from the food you did eat.

THE WATER DIET

The Water Diet is a diet plan you'll probably never see advertised, because it's too easy and everybody can already do it at home. But it sure works! In a German study, people were asked to drink two glasses of cold water, and then their metabolic rate was measured. Right away, it began to rise. Participants' metabolic rate rose an average of 30 percent and stayed that way for more than an hour. Drink eight glasses a day—real water, not some "watery" substitute— and you can count on burning off an extra 10 pounds a year. Drink it cold, too; not only does it taste better but your body has to burn extra calories to bring the temperature of the water up to body temperature—98.6 degrees.

Substituting water for caloric drinks is the single easiest way to reduce your daily calories, because it requires no changes in meals or other habits. The only resistance to this idea comes from people who think they don't like the taste of water. To them, I say, It's been too long since you tasted a pure, delicious glass of the stuff.

We are lucky enough to live in a country with an abundant supply of good water. For the majority of the world, that's a rarity. To them, it seems miraculous that in virtually any home in the United States someone can open a tap and get an endless stream of clean, safe drinking water. Yet we often take this for granted. Pretend you come from a place where clean water is scarce the next time you pour yourself a sparkling glass. Lift it to your lips and try to savor it for the first time. Ahhh!

Before I get too romantic, let's face facts: Some of us really do have bad-tasting water in our homes. Maybe your city water is heavily chlorinated. Maybe you live in Florida and have a high sulfur content in your water, which produces that rotten-egg smell. If that's the case, then no, I'm not going to make you drink it. A whole world of bottled waters awaits you. The mineral springs of Italy, France, Maine, and many other pristine spots sit gurgling on your supermarket shelves, each full of life-giving goodness.

Of course, if you drink nothing but bottled water, that will cost you a few bucks a week, and for some people this is a sticking point. Why should I pay for water, they think, when I can get a *real drink* for the same price? "A real drink" means soda, juice, energy drinks—something a company had to *make*, rather than just hold empty bottles in a spring until full. The bargain shopper in all of us kicks in. It's a great habit to have, but in this case it doesn't serve us well.

A better mentality to have—and it applies to a lot more than just drinks—is to stop thinking about food and drink purchases as buying *product* and to start thinking about them as buying *health*. That's why you eat, after all—to sustain life and health. Changing this thought process can be an incredibly simple yet powerful tool for altering your eating habits. Suddenly, that one-dollar liter of water seems like an incredible bargain. Half a day's worth of weight loss, plus hydration, improved energy, and disease prevention, for only a buck!

Start thinking this way, and you'll be replacing soda with water in no time. If you miss the taste of soda at first, you won't for long. We all have an instinctual love for the subtle flavor of water, but too many of us lose this because we've developed such an overwhelming taste for sweet things. Stroll through the grocery store and see how many products contain sugar, corn syrup, fructose, or any other word ending in *ose*, which means sugar. Our drinks are sweetened, our soup is sweetened, our pasta sauce is sweetened, and our breakfast cereals are intensely sweetened. A little sweetness tastes good on the tongue, so companies know an easy way to make their products taste good is to dump some sugar into them. After years of eating this way, the lack of sugar in a food starts to taste weird to us. We learn to confuse sugar with flavor.

To make healthy eating come naturally, we need to reset our palates back to a state of nature, to relearn the art of savoring food for its built-in flavor. If you can succeed, and truly lose your taste for sweet things, you'll find that you consume hundreds fewer calories each day without even thinking about it. That's why my assignment for you is to drink eight glasses a day of water for the next six weeks. Each Day Page gives you water-glass icons to help remind you. (And, since you don't need water as a recipe suggestion each day this week, I'll suggest recipes for a variety of meals and styles in order to give you a taste of what's to come in the following five weeks.)

Scared to go cold turkey on the soda? Has a Coke can been an extension of your arm for as long as you can remember? If that's the case, try my three-step plan for kicking the soda habit:

1. Switch to diet soda or cut your juice with sparkling water. I'm not a huge fan of diet soda. Yes, it is calorie-free, which is great, but its artificial sweeteners contain chemicals that haven't been around long enough for us to know what happens to the body when one drinks loads of them for forty years. They're probably safe, and probably better for you than sugar, but you never know. More important, if you drink diet sodas, you encourage your sweet tooth. You may not get the calories with the soda, but you're still conditioning yourself to crave the doughnuts and cookies of the world. If you guzzle diet soda, you'll never appreciate a grapefruit.

Try mixing half a glass of juice or an energy drink with an equal proportion of sparkling water. You'll get a better-tasting drink with half the calories. You can still consume a fair amount of calories this way, but it's a good halfway house for eliminating your sweet tooth.

2. **Drink pure sparkling water.** Keep increasing your ratio of sparkling water to juice until you are ready to drink the sparkling water straight up. If you're switching from diet soda, start by substituting one or two glasses a day of water for the soda; then gradually switch over to water entirely.

3. **Drink still water.** This step is optional. There are no health differences between sparkling and still water, but you get an extra dose of independence if you can break your reliance on store-bought water. Being able to have a glass of water anywhere you go sure makes things easy. It also saves you money. And really, in most of the United States, it couldn't be safer.

STRATEGIES FOR DRINKING MORE WATER

- Drink herbal tea. What is herbal tea but water with a little innocuous flavoring? Herbal tea is just as good for you as water (maybe better, because herbs such as chamomile have a natural relaxing effect) and tastes great.
- Drink decaf coffee and tea. Don't overdose on the high-test stuff—too much caffeine can stress you out—but drink as much decaf as you want. With coffee, make sure it's the Swiss water process for decaf, as this doesn't contain chemicals.
- Keep a fresh supply of water close at hand. Setting an attractive pitcher full of water someplace obvious, such as your desk, is like a daylong reminder to drink more water. Making your pitcher and glass beautiful helps "sweeten" the task!
- Keep bottles of water everywhere you spend a lot of time, so one is always within reach. Your living room, bedroom, car, and desk are good places to start.
- If your water doesn't taste good on its own, liven it up with a squeeze of lemon juice or a splash of rose water. Float a handful of lemon slices in your pitcher of water to make it beautiful *and* tasty.
- Drink skim milk. I adore skim milk! By drinking it, you kill two birds with one stone: It counts as a glass of water; plus, it's full of protein, calcium, and vitamins A and D. All for just 86 calories per glass! Don't substitute *all* your water-drinking for skim milk, or you'd be imbibing seven hundred calories a day. Drink a glass or two a day and think of it as a delicious, healthy snack.

The Intentional Eating Habit
Date_____

WEEK 1   MONDAY

Mission: Say Grace

Let's start off your six weeks with the easiest mission of all—but maybe the most important. Give thanks before a meal in whatever way feels right to you today. Then try to make it a daily habit every day of the program. Notice how much more enjoyable any activity is when you are completely present while doing it.

Mission Accomplished? ✓_____

WALK BOX

HOW FAR? _____ *1 mile* _____

STRENGTH TRAINING? _____ *No* _____

HOW'D IT GO? _____ *Very Fun Very Fast* _____

FOOD FOCUS: PASTA

SUGGESTED RECIPES

Fusilli with Smoked Turkey and
Roasted Veggies (p. 210)

Ravioli in Pumpkin Cream Sauce
 with Cranberries and Walnuts (p. 212)

BREAKFAST _Oatmeal/Pecan_   **LUNCH** Pasta/Turkey SALAD

DINNER Bean + Bacon Soup   **SNACKS** No
Salad / tbsp Ranch

DRINKS Water / Tonic/lime **DESSERTS** No

WATER 1 2 3 4 5 6 7 8

NOTES

The Intentional Eating Habit   Date_____

WEEK 1   TUESDAY

Mission: Get Hungry

Today, do something we rarely do in America. Get really and truly hungry. When that feeling of hunger first comes upon you, recognize it. Just be with it for a while. Externalize it. Say to yourself, Oh, so this is me experiencing hunger. Why panic? You're not going to die. You're not even going to faint. You'll get to food in a little while. You know it'll be there—it's everywhere!—and it will taste all the better for your having let yourself get good and hungry first. In the meantime, you've taken control of something you thought you simply had to respond to.

Mission Accomplished? ___✓___

WALK BOX

HOW FAR? _2miles Video_____

STRENGTH TRAINING? _Snow blowing_____

HOW'D IT GO? _Very Good_____

FOOD FOCUS: HEALTHY MAIN DISHES

SUGGESTED RECIPES

Cumin and Orange–Scented Pork Loin (p. 225)

Turkey Picadillo (p. 222)

BREAKFAST 1 cup shredded
wheat w/ 12 almonds

LUNCH ½ cup Pasta salad w/turkey
1 grilled cheese

DINNER _____

SNACKS _____

DRINKS Water 2 cups Coffe

DESSERTS 1 Sugarfre popcicle

WATER 1 2 3 4 5 6 7 8

NOTES

_____
_____
_____
_____
_____
_____
_____
_____
_____
_____
_____
_____
_____
_____

The Intentional Eating Habit   Date_____

WEEK 1   WEDNESDAY

Mission: Food Is Not Love

Today, don't worry about anything but your emotional state as you eat. (Believe me, that's plenty!) Before each meal, snack, or treat, ask yourself, How do I feel? What am I hoping to get from this food? If the answer is that you feel hungry and you're hoping to get full and energized, go right ahead and eat. If the answer is that you're feeling sad, lonely, or bored, then put that food away and go for a walk. A walk is the very best substitute for emotional eating because it makes false hunger disappear and leaves you upbeat and energized. Use it as your solution to emotional eating in the future.

Mission Accomplished? ___✓___

WALK BOX

HOW FAR? _____

STRENGTH TRAINING? _____

HOW'D IT GO? _____

FOOD FOCUS: SURPRISING SALADS

SUGGESTED RECIPES

Black Bean, Orange, and Cucumber Salad (p. 197)

Surprise Beet-Mango Salad (p. 197)

BREAKFAST _1 Cup Shredded Wheat_ LUNCH_____

_1 Banana_____ _____

DINNER_____ SNACKS_____

_____ _____

DRINKS_____ DESSERTS_____

_____ _____

WATER 1 2 3 4 5 6 7 8

NOTES

The Intentional Eating Habit

WEEK 1   THURSDAY

Mission: Food Is Not Background Music

I'm sorry to say that your munching days are over—at least for today. Confine your eating today to specific meals. A snack is fine, but it must be small and eaten in ten minutes or less—no grazing. Having times that are for eating and times that aren't is a great way to train your body not to crave food constantly. So, no eating at work, in the car, in the living room, in the movie theater, or in bed. If your evening TV viewing needs a steady trickle of food, then maybe it's time to improve the quality of your entertainment!

Mission Accomplished? _____

WALK BOX

HOW FAR? _____

STRENGTH TRAINING? _____

HOW'D IT GO? _____

FOOD FOCUS: FRIENDLY VEGGIES

SUGGESTED RECIPES

Zucchini Surprise Fries (p. 227)

Sesame Green Beans (p. 228)

BREAKFAST_____ LUNCH_____

_____ _____

DINNER_____ SNACKS_____

_____ _____

DRINKS_____ DESSERTS_____

_____ _____

WATER 1 2 3 4 5 6 7 8

NOTES

_____

_____

_____

_____

_____

_____

_____

_____

_____

_____

_____

_____

_____

The Intentional Eating Habit   Date_____

WEEK 1   FRIDAY

Mission: If It Doesn't Taste Good, Don't Eat It

Some taste specialists claim that after the first three or four bites of something, you don't really taste it. There's some truth to this. That first bite is the one that really socks you with flavors bursting in your mouth. Soon, though, just as you stop hearing a steady noise after a few minutes, you're eating on memory. Maybe you still register a basic sweetness or saltiness, but not much more. Think about this as you eat today, and keep eating only if you are truly enjoying it. You don't get special credit for finishing anything—in fact, you get special credit if you *don't*.

Mission Accomplished? _____

WALK BOX

HOW FAR? _____

STRENGTH TRAINING? _____

HOW'D IT GO? _____

FOOD FOCUS: LIVELY RICE

SUGGESTED RECIPES

Cajun Red Beans and Rice (p. 233)

Coconut Rice (p. 233)

BREAKFAST_____ LUNCH_____

_____ _____

DINNER_____ SNACKS_____

_____ _____

DRINKS_____ DESSERTS_____

_____ _____

WATER 1 2 3 4 5 6 7 8

NOTES

_____

_____

_____

_____

_____

_____

_____

_____

_____

_____

_____

_____

The Intentional Eating Habit   Date_____

WEEK 1   SATURDAY

Mission: Eat for the Future

Eat a very healthy breakfast or lunch today, something with a nice mix of protein, carbs, and fat. Then note how you feel an hour later. (Put a reminder somewhere, even in your day planner, so you remember to do this.) Now here's the fun part: Do the opposite with another meal today. Eat something nice and greasy, like fast food, or just straight refined carbs, like a bagel. Then monitor how you feel an hour later. That grumpy, low-energy, distracted, shaky feeling is the clearest indicator that your body isn't happy with the second choice. Maturing in our eating habits, tuning in to the fact that food affects us not just at the moment when chip hits tongue but for hours afterward, will help us get the most pleasure *and* health from our diet.

Mission Accomplished? _____

WALK BOX

HOW FAR? _____

STRENGTH TRAINING? _____

HOW'D IT GO? _____

FOOD FOCUS: FRUIT CONCOCTIONS

SUGGESTED RECIPES

Guava Granita (p. 239)

Cranberry-Orange Turkey Sandwich (p. 195)

BREAKFAST_____   LUNCH_____
_____   _____

DINNER_____   SNACKS_____
_____   _____

DRINKS_____   DESSERTS_____
_____

WATER [1] [2] [3] [4] [5] [6] [7] [8]

NOTES

_____

_____

_____

_____

_____

_____

_____

_____

_____

_____

_____

_____

The Intentional Eating Habit   Date_____

WEEK 1   SUNDAY WRAP-UP

THE PERFECT SUPPORT SYSTEM

PLANNING
Three smart behaviors I can adopt next week to support my eating goals:
1. _____
2. _____
3. _____

EDUCATION
What I've learned so far:

NEW HABITS   FOOD SOLUTIONS
Intentional Eating   Water

REPETITION
This week's behaviors:
(Put a ✓ next to those you'll keep doing, an X next to those that weren't useful to you, and an → next to those that you'll try again later.)

1. ___ Say Grace
2. ___ Get Hungry
3. ___ Food Is Not Love
4. ___ Food Is Not Background Music
5. ___ If It Doesn't Taste Good, Don't Eat It
6. ___ Eat for the Future

Other Intentional Eating Habits you thought of this week: _____
_____
_____
_____
_____

FLEXIBILITY

Three ways I can make these habits work better for me:

1. _____
2. _____
3. _____

EXERCISE

Miles/steps walked this week: _____
_____

Other exercise: _____
_____
_____

CELEBRATION!

Three things I'm grateful for this week:

1. _____
2. _____
3. _____

TRANSFORMATION

I surprised myself this week by: _____

NOTES

_____
_____
_____
_____
_____
_____
_____

8. Week 2
The Breakfast Habit

Here's a recipe for disaster: Take a child, fill her up with orange juice and frosted flakes, and send her out the door. Here's another: Take yourself, pick up a bagel and coffee for breakfast, then head to work.

You can shuffle these variables and still end up with the same bad formula. Substitute any other kind of juice or soda for the orange juice, and any other sugary breakfast cereal, Pop-Tart, muffin, or doughnut for the frosted flakes or bagel. Any way you cut it, what you have is a person starting the day with a sugar rush that is going to come crashing down in about an hour, leaving her irritated, unable to concentrate, and *hungry*.

Breakfast has become a carbfest in this country, and it's setting us up for trouble. Breakfast is the meal where you break your nightlong fast; what you eat first in the morning sets the tone for your whole day. As I explained earlier when discussing nutrition in chapter 3 (and will do in more detail in this week's Food Focus), eating a meal that is mostly refined carbohydrates, whether sugars or starches, begins a roller coaster of rising and falling sugar levels in your blood, leaving you constantly craving more carbs, which leads to weight gain and, eventually, diabetes.

Skipping breakfast, the other increasingly common practice, is even worse. After a night of sleep, your metabolism is low and needs the cue of food to signal it to rev up its engines. If you don't eat, your metabolism stays stuck in neutral. By burning fewer calories throughout the day, not only will you have less energy and creativity but you can actually gain weight. That's right: Eating a decent breakfast can help you maintain a normal weight, as well as make you a more productive and pleasant person.

When I think back on how we became a nation of breakfast sugar eaters, I trace the development back to the 1980s. With more couples working two jobs, morning time was at a premium. Breakfast became a fend-for-yourself, no-cook, fifteen-minute meal. The only foods that fit that description were cold cereals and bread products.

The low-fat, anticholesterol craze was also in full swing in the 1980s, which meant the egg was out. Eggs are high in cholesterol and have some fat. Staple breakfast fare for decades, they are also packed with protein and vitamins. We didn't know it then, but we now know that the cholesterol in them doesn't affect your body's blood-cholesterol level. Jettisoning eggs for low-fat sugary cereals at breakfast inadvertently helped obesity, diabetes, and heart disease rates spiral out of control, all the while creating a country of workers, students, and drivers who couldn't concentrate without eating a candy bar at 10:00 AM.

Eggs are just the most obvious example of the kinds of food we need to start eating again for breakfast. Eating a mix of protein, fats, and carbs at breakfast fills us up with food that is slowly digested by the body, meaning we stay full and alert, concentrating on our job or studies instead of dreaming about lunch. The carbs give us energy, the protein helps us concentrate, and the fat keeps us full for hours.

Once you understand this, you'll see why I think we need to forget everything we've learned about what are and are not "breakfast foods." We've got it all backward. The typical American pattern is to eat little or no breakfast, a medium lunch, and a huge dinner. This gives us an energy deficit in the morning, when we least need it, and a massive calorie load in the evening, when we are least likely to burn it off. (Instead, any unburned calories get converted into fat.) Start doing it the other way around. Remember my favorite saying: Eat breakfast like a king, lunch like a queen, and dinner like a pauper.

What constitutes a kingly breakfast? This week's suggestions will get you started.

SIX STRATEGIES FOR DEVELOPING YOUR BREAKFAST HABIT

1. PROTEIN POWER

Why protein for breakfast? Because it isn't carbs! The body takes longer to break down protein, meaning you stay full longer and won't get spikes in blood-sugar levels. Unsaturated fat is fine for breakfast, too, but you need something solid to put it on, which boils down to protein or carbs. Generally, by eating a mix of all three nutrients, you assure yourself of maintaining high energy until lunch. Eggs are the classic breakfast source of protein, but don't forget natural peanut butter. Breakfast meats like bacon and sausage, as well as cheese, tend to be high in saturated fat, so use them sparingly. Deli meats are better. Smoked salmon is a good source of protein, though it's high in sodium. What about beans, nuts, low-fat milk, yogurt, or cottage cheese? See what creations you can come up with.

2. Break the Social Rules

"You're eating *that* for breakfast?" I have a friend whose favorite breakfast is dinner leftovers, and that's the refrain he usually hears whenever he sticks Chinese takeout or lasagne in the microwave at eight o'clock in the morning. He used to do it surreptitiously, so as not to face the judgment of what does and does not constitute socially acceptable breakfast food, but now he's over that. He knows how much better he feels when he eats a balanced meal for breakfast, so he doesn't care what anyone else thinks. Break free of social judgment and determine just what it is you really want to eat each morning. Whether it's chicken salad, tacos, or gumbo, you go right ahead. You'll have yourself to thank later on.

3. Coffee Is Not Breakfast

Don't make the mistake of thinking coffee gives you more energy in the morning. It might help wake you up, but caffeine is just an accelerant. It takes whatever energy you already have and burns it faster. Your heart beats faster and you feel more alert, but you also run out of energy more quickly. That's why you feel that slump a couple of hours after drinking caffeine. While coffee may be the spark you use to get your engine started, make sure you fill up your tank, too.

4. Get Wholesome

As you'll learn in this week's Food Focus, whole grains are digested much more slowly by the body than simple starches like white bread or potatoes, so they keep you full a lot longer on the same amount of calories. That's why they're a key part of your weight-loss goal, and there's no better time to have them than at breakfast, when many of us find their mild flavor and rich warmth so comforting.

Nutritionists pay a lot of attention to whole grains, telling people why they need to eat more of them, but they rarely explain that the way those grains are processed makes a huge difference in their health benefits. Even whole wheat can cause a surge in blood sugar if it's ground so fine that your body can absorb it right away. The coarser the grind, the longer your stomach needs to work on it. Take oatmeal. A lot of people have been told to eat oatmeal to lower their cholesterol and blood pressure, so they open a package of instant oatmeal every morning. But what do you think makes that oatmeal instant? It's because the company has precooked it and ground it so finely that the grains can absorb water right away. That same fineness allows your blood to absorb those carbs as soon as you eat them. A great rule to keep in mind is that the longer it takes a grain to cook, the slower it will be digested. We all can afford the one-minute investment in our health by cooking quick oats (which are chopped up but not pulverized) rather than instant, and really I don't know anyone who can't take the five minutes to cook the old-fashioned oats (which are rolled but not chopped) instead of the instant. If you have leisurely mornings, you might want to try steel-cut oats, which are the coarsest of all. They take twenty minutes in the pot (less if you soak them the night before) but provide an unparalleled nutty taste and chewy texture, and provoke the lowest insulin response of all.

5. DRINK YOUR BREAKFAST

The latest trend in breakfasts is high-protein drinks, which usually contain a mixture of soy-based protein, sugars or sugar substitutes, and flavorings. These can work pretty well. They give you a nice mix of protein and carbs, as well as plenty of energy and vitamins to get you through the first half of the day. One warning, though: If they constitute your entire breakfast, you might still end up snacking. That's because, as researchers are learning, the body *wants* to chew. Regardless of what's consumed, the very act of chewing helps the body feel satisfied. Along with your protein drink, you might want to have a piece of fruit or whole-grain toast to give your jaw (and stomach) something to work on. And don't forget that you can concoct lots of delicious protein drinks on your own. A fruit smoothie made with fresh berries and low-fat yogurt packs all the protein punch of that powdered soy drink and tastes a whole lot better.

6. DELAY BREAKFAST

Already I can hear the chorus of resistance. Lots of you out there are saying, "But, Leslie, I can't stand the sight of food when I first wake up. There's no way I'm choking down even a muffin, much less a turkey sandwich." That's all right; we can work with that. For you breakfast dreaders, it's fine to stick to coffee when you wake up, then eat your first meal at ten o'clock or whenever you feel ready. Just plan accordingly so that, when you do eat, you follow the healthy guidelines suggested above and schedule your other meals sensibly. Breakfast at 10:00, lunch at 3:00, and dinner at 8:00 may work best for you. If so, go for it. Flexing your plan to suit your style will be a key component of your success.

Whole Grains and Legumes

My teenage daughter does a lot of homework. I want her grades to be as good as possible, so am I ever tempted to do her homework for her? Of course not. I might give her a pointer or two, but I know that doing the work herself is important. The same is true with my older relatives. Sure, I'll help out if they can't physically do something, but the more they can continue to do things on their own and be independent, the stronger they'll be. We were all meant to be physically and mentally active. The more we stick with that, the healthier we are.

My body is the same. It's designed to do physical work, and also to work on its food. The machines that now do much of the work of breaking down food for us—that strip the hulls off the grains and crush the kernels into powder, or refine the sugars out of the sugarcane, or even boil the potato into a soft mash—are all relatively recent arrivals on the scene. You have a stomach capable of taking a tough lump of meat and liquefying it in a matter of minutes, so with that kind of power at your disposal, why not use it?

Your entire digestive system is a fantastic arrangement for getting energy and nutrition out of food. First your teeth chop up the food into manageable pieces. Then your stomach attacks the food with a combination of water, acid, and powerful muscular contractions that smash it up. When it's done, the liquefied food is sent to the small intestine, which picks all the nutrients out and transfers them to the bloodstream.

This system is necessary because foods in their natural state don't usually give up their nutrients easily. It takes a lot of work to get through the tough skins and hulls of plant foods before reaching the good stuff. But that's okay—our bodies are up to the task.

The main nutrient that our bodies are after is carbohydrates, the sugars that power our muscles. And the problem actually comes when our bodies have too easy a time getting these sugars. Every form of carbohydrate, from cotton candy to grapes, white bread, and carrots, gets broken down into the same sugar molecule. What's different is how long it takes the body to do this, and what else (such as fiber and vitamins) is included in the package.

With cotton candy, or soda, or even white bread, nothing else is included. It's just sugar, straight up (starches are simply many sugar molecules strung together), and you may as well inject it into your veins yourself, it takes so little time to get into your bloodstream. If you're familiar with diabetes, you know what happens next. That huge spike in blood-sugar levels causes your pancreas to pump out insulin, the hormone that acts like a key to "unlock" your muscle cells and push the sugar into them. But when the spike in blood-sugar levels is strong and quick enough, you get a wild seesaw effect. Your pancreas creates so much insulin to deal with the blood sugar that it deals with it too well. By the time the flood of insulin has finished with the blood sugar, it has pushed so much sugar out of your blood that you end up with low blood sugar—hypoglycemia. That low blood sugar signals your brain to grab more food fast—especially some carbs to get that blood sugar back to normal quickly. Soon you're eating carbs every few hours, feeling briefly satisfied, and then quickly becoming ravenous for more.

*Every form of carbohydrate, from
cotton candy to grapes,
white bread, and carrots, gets
broken down into the same
sugar molecule.*

This is the rationale behind low-carb diets. Avoid the carbs and you no longer get the peaks in blood sugar and the accompanying valleys. When it comes to avoiding soda and white bread, this theory is absolutely right.

But the baby gets thrown out with the bathwater when some of these diets recommend avoiding more complex forms of carbohydrates as well. Whole-wheat flour is the pure-carb white flour (which would have been the "starter fuel" for the wheat seed when it grew) wrapped in its original husk of fiber, good fat, a little protein, and vitamins. Your body wants that starter fuel, and it gets it, but it takes a lot longer to break through the fibrous husk to do so. As a result, you digest the carbs from whole grains more slowly—as it was meant to be.

What about the other stuff? The protein goes to build new muscle, while the vitamins and fat help keep a number of body processes running smoothly. The fiber is essential to health, as well. Fiber can't be digested by the body, which sounds like trouble, but again, that's how it's supposed to be. Some fiber acts like a bowling ball, keeping your digestive system clear of obstructions. Other fiber absorbs water and binds with cholesterol-forming fat, meaning these artery-clogging compounds never make it into your bloodstream. That's why the butter in your oatmeal is less likely to cause cardiovascular disease than the butter on your white toast (and why a diet high in fiber helps you lose weight by absorbing fewer calories from your food).

You get no fiber with refined carbs like white flour and white rice. You also don't get many vitamins. Some of the vitamins removed when wheat flour is refined into white are vitamin E, vitamin B_6, magnesium, manganese, riboflavin, niacin, zinc, potassium, thiamin, iron, and phosphorus. Small amounts of protein and healthy fat complete the picture of what doesn't make the final cut with white flour.

Still not convinced you should switch to whole grains? Then let me make an argument in favor of flavor. Whole wheat, brown rice, and other whole grains have a rich, buttery, nutty taste that refined grains can't match. We think we prefer the soft tastelessness of white rice and flour only because that's what we grew up with. It's familiar. Once you acquire a taste for the goodness of whole grains, you'll never go back.

In a way, beans are like giant grains, which is why they are often grouped together. Like grains, they are plant seeds that make excellent human food when cooked. They offer many of the same benefits: lots of fiber and vitamins along with the carbs. Unlike grains, beans are also a great source of protein. Whether you prefer black beans, kidney beans, chickpeas, or peas, you are getting one of the world's perfect foods. And at only pennies per pound, they are truly supplying health at basement prices!

Beans and whole grains actually make a perfect nutritional team. Unlike animal protein, the protein in legumes doesn't provide all the essential amino acids humans need for health—unless you combine it with whole grains to make what's called a "perfect protein." This is why they show up together in the traditional cooking of so many cultures—beans and corn in Mexico and Latin America, chickpeas and couscous in North Africa, rice and soybeans in Asia.

The drawback to natural grains and legumes is the time it takes to cook them: forty-five minutes for brown rice, hours for dried beans. How often do you walk into your kitchen hours ahead of time to plan your meal? I don't do that, either. Fortunately, there are plenty of shortcuts we can take. Instant brown rice that cooks in ten minutes is available. With beans or chickpeas, the solution is to use canned beans, which are already cooked. You can have Cajun beans and rice or a quick vegetable chili ready in less than thirty minutes. You can also make brown rice a day or two in advance, store it in the fridge, and reheat as needed. It tastes just as good.

STRATEGIES FOR GETTING MORE WHOLE GRAINS AND LEGUMES

- Choose oatmeal, multigrain pancakes, or whole-grain cold cereals for breakfast.
- Switch all your bread to multigrain breads that list whole wheat and other grains or seeds in the ingredients list before simple "wheat flour."
- Use whole-wheat tortillas, piecrusts, and bagels.
- Instead of potato chips, snack on all-natural stone-ground tortilla chips.

- Use canned beans for convenience.
- Throw out your white rice and use only brown from now on. Use the regular kind, which cooks in forty-five minutes, when possible, but have some instant on hand for when you need a fast meal.

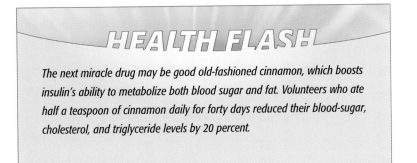

HEALTH FLASH

The next miracle drug may be good old-fashioned cinnamon, which boosts insulin's ability to metabolize both blood sugar and fat. Volunteers who ate half a teaspoon of cinnamon daily for forty days reduced their blood-sugar, cholesterol, and triglyceride levels by 20 percent.

The Breakfast Habit

WEEK 2   MONDAY

Mission: Protein Power

Today, you will banish the morning blues from your life. Once you have a high-protein breakfast and notice how this produces a high-powered morning, you'll never go back to Crispy Crunch. Eggs in any form are my top choice, but try natural peanut butter, yogurt with nuts and fruit, or a healthy cut of meat. And don't forget this week's Food Focus. Try to have some whole-grain toast with that.

Mission Accomplished? _____

WALK BOX

HOW FAR? _____

STRENGTH TRAINING? _____

HOW'D IT GO? _____

FOOD FOCUS: THE INCREDIBLE, EDIBLE EGG

SUGGESTED RECIPES

Spinach and Chèvre Omelette (p. 194)

Fried Eggs on Garlic Toast (p. 193)

BREAKFAST_____ LUNCH_____

_____ _____

DINNER_____ SNACKS_____

_____ _____

DRINKS_____ DESSERTS_____

_____ _____

WATER

1 2 3 4 5 6 7 8

NOTES

_____

_____

_____

_____

_____

_____

_____

_____

_____

_____

_____

_____

WEEK 2   TUESDAY

Mission: Break the Social Rules

Why is it that we let other people tell us what's acceptable breakfast fare—even when other people aren't around? A breakfast sandwich (meat, egg, and cheese on bread) is breakfast, yet a ham sandwich (meat and cheese on bread) isn't? The sad thing is, so many dinners, with their emphasis on protein and vegetables, make perfect breakfasts. Today, throw social constraint to the wind and have something *crazy* for breakfast. Leftovers work great. Chicken breast? Burritos? You pick. Do half-sized portions if you don't like eating a lot of food in the morning.

Mission Accomplished? _____

WALK BOX

HOW FAR? _____

STRENGTH TRAINING? _____

HOW'D IT GO? _____

FOOD FOCUS: RADICAL BREAKFASTS

SUGGESTED RECIPES

Chicken Aloha (p. 223)

Southwest Black Bean Fritters (p. 232)

BREAKFAST_____ LUNCH_____

_____ _____

DINNER_____ SNACKS_____

_____ _____

DRINKS_____ DESSERTS_____

_____ _____

WATER ⛁ 1 ⛁ 2 ⛁ 3 ⛁ 4 ⛁ 5 ⛁ 6 ⛁ 7 ⛁ 8

NOTES

_____

_____

_____

_____

_____

_____

_____

_____

_____

_____

_____

_____

_____

The Breakfast Habit   Date_____

Mission: Coffee Is Not Breakfast

Today will be an easy day for you if you are a good breakfast eater. If not, it will be step one in making a marked difference in your health, energy, and waistline. If you generally have nothing but a cup of coffee, start small. Even a bowl of cold cereal with skim milk will at least help your metabolism kick in. Oatmeal with skim milk and raisins is better—a nice mix of complex carbs, protein, and fiber. An egg with whole-grain toast is better still.

Mission Accomplished? _____

WALK BOX

HOW FAR? _____

STRENGTH TRAINING? _____

HOW'D IT GO? _____

FOOD FOCUS: EASY DOES IT

SUGGESTED RECIPES

Cinnamon-Walnut Muffins (p. 190)

Broiled Grapefruit with Cinnamon (p. 244)

BREAKFAST_____ LUNCH_____

_____ _____

DINNER_____ SNACKS_____

_____ _____

DRINKS_____ DESSERTS_____

_____ _____

WATER ① ② ③ ④ ⑤ ⑥ ⑦ ⑧

NOTES

_____

_____

_____

_____

_____

_____

_____

_____

_____

_____

_____

_____

The Breakfast Habit Date_____

WEEK 2   THURSDAY

Mission: Get Wholesome

Instead of that white-flour bagel, choose whole-wheat or multigrain bread and notice how much better you feel an hour later. Many breakfast cereals are now made completely with whole grains, but the other thing to keep in mind is how finely milled the grains are. Cheerios are made from whole grain, but it has been pulverized to powder, meaning your body still digests the grain much more quickly than the grain in cereals like All-Bran or Special K. But all breakfast cereals are finely ground enough to cause a pretty strong insulin response, so old-fashioned oatmeal or granola (see recipe page 190) is a better choice. See how coarse you can go at breakfast, and plan on making white flour a thing of your past.

Mission Accomplished? _____

WALK BOX

HOW FAR? _____

STRENGTH TRAINING? _____

HOW'D IT GO? _____

FOOD FOCUS: WHOLE GRAINS

SUGGESTED RECIPES

Cranberry-Almond Granola (p. 190)

Nutty Pancakes (p. 191)

84   *Leslie Sansone's Eat Smart, Walk Strong*

BREAKFAST_____ LUNCH_____

_____ _____

DINNER_____ SNACKS_____

_____ _____

DRINKS_____ DESSERTS_____

_____ _____

WATER 1 2 3 4 5 6 7 8

NOTES

_____

_____

_____

_____

_____

_____

_____

_____

_____

_____

_____

_____

The Breakfast Habit   Date_____

WEEK 2   FRIDAY

Mission: Drink Your Breakfast

If you are one of those people who finds the idea of choking down an omelette in the morning pure torture, breakfast shakes may be the answer. You still get to have your toast in the morning, while your protein and vitamins go down in a delicious drink. You can even drink it on your way to work if you prefer. Yogurt smoothies are easy and versatile, but if you want a change of pace, try a soy shake.

Mission Accomplished? _____

WALK BOX

HOW FAR? _____

STRENGTH TRAINING? _____

HOW'D IT GO? _____

FOOD FOCUS: SMOOTHIES

SUGGESTED RECIPES

Blueberry Breakfast Smoothie (p. 189)

Orange Mango Smoothie (p. 189)

BREAKFAST_____   LUNCH_____

_____   _____

DINNER_____   SNACKS_____

_____   _____

DRINKS_____   DESSERTS_____

_____   _____

WATER   1   2   3   4   5   6   7   8

NOTES

_____

_____

_____

_____

_____

_____

_____

_____

_____

_____

_____

_____

_____

The Breakfast Habit   Date_____

Mission: Delay Breakfast

It's 8:00 AM and you know you're supposed to eat something healthy, but really all you want is to be left alone with your coffee and the paper for half an hour. Fine. I wouldn't want to deny anybody their simple pleasures. That coffee will get you through the first couple hours of your day anyway. But I also don't want to see that morning slump, so plan on a midmorning snack for breakfast today. If you spend your days out of the house, take a healthy muffin with you, or plan on grabbing some eggs somewhere. If you're at home, you have more options. Either way, see how changing up your routine makes you much more aware of your body and its needs.

Mission Accomplished? _____

WALK BOX

HOW FAR? _____

STRENGTH TRAINING? _____

HOW'D IT GO? _____

FOOD FOCUS: MIDMORNING SNACK

SUGGESTED RECIPES

Spanish Tuna and Chickpea Salad (p. 198)

Oatmeal-Raisin Chocolate Chip Cookies (p. 241)

BREAKFAST_____ LUNCH_____

_____ _____

DINNER_____ SNACKS_____

_____ _____

DRINKS_____ DESSERTS_____

_____ _____

WATER 1 2 3 4 5 6 7 8

NOTES

_____

_____

_____

_____

_____

_____

_____

_____

_____

_____

_____

_____

_____

The Breakfast Habit Date_____

WEEK 2 SUNDAY WRAP-UP

THE PERFECT SUPPORT SYSTEM

PLANNING
Three smart behaviors I can adopt next week to support my eating goals:
1. _____
2. _____
3. _____

EDUCATION
What I've learned so far:

NEW HABITS	FOOD SOLUTIONS
Intentional Eating	Water
Breakfast	Whole Grains and Legumes

REPETITION
This week's behaviors:
(Put a ✓ next to those you'll keep doing, an X next to those that weren't useful to you, and an ➤ next to those that you'll try again later.)
1. ___ Protein Power
2. ___ Break the Social Rules
3. ___ Coffee Is Not Breakfast
4. ___ Get Wholesome
5. ___ Drink Your Breakfast
6. ___ Delay Breakfast

Other Breakfast Habits you thought of this week:

_____

_____

Two behaviors from the past two weeks that are becoming habits:

1. _____

2. _____

90   *Leslie Sansone's Eat Smart, Walk Strong*

FLEXIBILITY

Three ways I can make these habits work better for me:

1. _____
2. _____
3. _____

EXERCISE

Miles/steps walked this week: _____

_____

Other exercise: _____

_____

_____

CELEBRATION!

Three things I'm grateful for this week:

1. _____
2. _____
3. _____

TRANSFORMATION

I surprised myself this week by: _____

NOTES

_____

_____

_____

_____

_____

_____

_____

9. Week 3
The Portion-Control Habit

You are going to be amazed at the tremendous impact this week's simple practices have on your waistline. I call this the "no-brainer" week: Some of the solutions sound obvious, but what isn't obvious is the way most of us squirm out of employing these solutions to solve our weight problems. We usually don't do these easy things. Make them a habit, starting this week, and you have won half the battle.

The secret to the portion-control habit is the delay that exists between when we eat and when we feel full. It's about fifteen minutes—the time it takes for the first wave of food to pass from the stomach into the beginning of the small intestine. There, chemical messengers sense the food and send signals to the brain, saying, "We got it. All set here. You can stop eating now." Then your brain turns off the hunger switch.

Unfortunately, there are a few glitches with this system. One is that we can put away quite a few extra calories in the fifteen minutes it takes to receive those first "all full" signals. Another glitch is that our "hungry" signals can be so strong that it takes some very loud "too full!" messages from the small intestine to finally stop us from eating. Basically, we get so hungry, and the food tastes so good, we get on a roll and can't stop. Once we finally do heed the pleading of the small intestine, we still face another fifteen minutes of food we've already eaten working its way from the stomach to the intestine, which means another fifteen minutes of "Turn it off. Turn it off!" messages. You know the feeling: the after-dinner "I can't believe I ate the whole thing" bloat.

Learning to turn off the eating switch a little early doesn't come automatically to anyone. Given the opportunity to overeat, most of us will. As I explained, for much of human history, scarce food was a more common problem than too much food, so the occasional bout of overeating was a pretty good survival mechanism. That's not true anymore, which is why cultivating the habit of eating limited portions is the new survival mechanism.

Now, let's face reality: You can't really count on your mind or body to help you out in this endeavor. At least not the mind or body confronted by a chocolate cake sitting inches away on the table. What you need to do is put your mind into action *before* the chocolate cake makes its dramatic appearance, and set things up so you run out of food before you've eaten too much. At first, your brain will be saying, More, more! I need more! But fifteen minutes later, you'll realize you were full after all. Once this becomes a habit, and you learn to recognize the flow of feelings, you won't notice that urgent desire to keep eating anymore. That's what habits are all about.

Running out of food at just the right time means learning what a portion size should be, giving yourself that much, and removing all possibilities to "supplement" that serving by sampling as you cook or eating the leftovers because "there isn't enough to put back." A table laden with serving bowls has a warm family feeling—and on Thanksgiving and special occasions, go for it—but it's an invitation to keep ladling a little more food onto your plate, until you've doubled your dinner.

That's the most obvious example, and it can be addressed by the "one and done" rule: You get a plate of food, and that is your meal. No seconds, no exceptions. Putting even the possibility of seconds out of your mind at the beginning of the meal will make you less tempted later on.

Ah, but the hungry little child who lives in us all has figured out a way around this one. "Okay, I'll take just one plateful, but I'm gonna use a plate the size of a trash-can lid!" You may think that you wouldn't fall for this, and maybe you wouldn't, but that would make you one of the rare few. In study after study, it has been shown that we eat and drink more from large dishes and containers than from small ones. We have it ingrained in us to eat what's given to us, not to waste. But when what's given to us is a megatub of popcorn, we'd do much better to waste it. Even if we quit halfway down, we've still eaten *four times* the popcorn served in the regular twelve-ounce boxes at movie theaters thirty years ago.

It's not just us, either. Studies of professional bartenders—people who pour drinks hundreds of times a day for a living—found that they wound up pouring more into wide glasses than into narrow ones, while estimating that they'd poured less.

(Which is why those huge balloon wineglasses so in vogue probably encourage excessive alcohol consumption.) Along with the American home and American car, the size of America's dishes is bulging at the seams. Think about your grandmother's glasses and dishes; I bet they were smaller than what you use.

Bottom line: Switching to smaller glassware and dishes is one of the easiest ways to send subtle cues to your brain to eat less. You'll end up serving yourself less without even realizing it.

But what you serve will indeed be a portion size. We have become so accustomed to the giant helpings in restaurants that seeing an official serving size can come as a shock. But that's all we really need. See the box on this page for a better sense of some common serving sizes.

Do those look like servings taken from your daughter's dollhouse? If so, it's not because you need more food than that, but because we've all gotten used to much larger portions. Starting in the seventies, the sizes of many of the common foods we eat began to get larger—*much* larger. And this growth has continued right up to the present. A study at New York University found that of 181 different food products, 180 had increased in size over the years (only a slice of bread remained the same). The size of a McDonald's french fry has more than tripled since the product was first introduced. Even the 1998 Supersize fries weren't large enough; by 2001, that size had become the "large" and the new Supersize was bigger still! The same thing has happened with sodas. Just look at the cup holder in a ten-year-old car; it won't even hold most of the drinks you buy in a convenience store today.

As part of its food-pyramid recommendations, the USDA offers a serving-size guide. But food manufacturers aren't listening. They offer us bagels that are 95 percent larger than a serving size, muffins that are 233 percent larger, pasta that is 380 percent larger, and cookies that are a whopping 600 percent larger than what we should have. When we buy a muffin, we don't think, How many servings is this? We just eat the muffin.

So food manufacturers get some of the blame for starting us down the road to

SERVING SIZE EQUIVALENTS

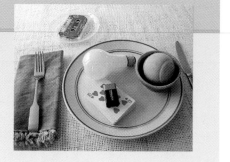

Meat:	Deck of cards
Potato, pasta, or rice:	Lightbulb
Fruit or vegetable:	Tennis ball
Butter, oil, or dressing:	9-volt battery
Dessert:	Cassette tape

overeating. But in a dog-eat-dog world, where they are all competing with one another to offer you better value for your money, it's hard to blame them. You need to take it upon yourself to know what a sensible portion is, no matter what gigantic candy bar comes your way. Following the advice in these six strategies will go a long way toward fulfilling this goal.

Six Strategies for Developing Your Portion-Control Habit

1. Perfect Portions

Take a little time to educate yourself on what a perfect portion size is for your size and activity level. You can visit the FDA Website at www.usda.org for the most up-to-date guidelines. To get a sense of what a typical meal should look like, refer again to the box on page 94.

2. Smaller Dishes

Not many of us put our dinner plate on a scale and carefully load it with exactly the right amount of food before eating. We just fill up a plate and call it dinner. If you switch to a plate that is 25 percent smaller, you'll eat 25 percent less. It's that simple! Don't worry about this leaving you hungry. Your new little plate isn't too small; the old one was too big. Finish your plate of food, walk away, and notice how you are perfectly full a few minutes later.

Don't believe me? Then consider this study. Researchers at Pennsylvania State University measured how many calories women consume at lunch. They found that doubling the size of the women's entrées caused the women to eat one hundred extra calories. Making the entrées richer (by adding cheese to pasta) caused the women to consume an additional 120 calories. And making the entrées both large and extra rich caused the women to consume an additional 220 calories. But the really shocking thing? These women didn't feel any more full than the women eating normal portions, and they didn't eat any less dinner that night!

3. Skinny Glasses

Don't underestimate the impact of drinks on your diet. As I discussed in chapter 7, the average American consumes 450 calories in liquids every day, which works out to a difference of forty-five pounds per year! Even if you don't want to give up your soda just yet, there is a more subtle game you can play. Switch to tall, thin glasses and you will drink less while enjoying it more. That's because we seem to have internal guidelines that monitor how much we've drunk by how far the line in our glass has dropped, regardless of total volume. Wrap up your short, fat glasses (or, worse, your tall and wide glasses!) and stick them in the basement. They weren't doing you any favors.

4. One and Done

So much of healthy eating is training your body what to expect. If we are used to going back for seconds, we almost always will, regardless of the size of our first helping. We'll even feel a false hunger as we anticipate that second plate of food. Instead, develop the habit of serving yourself whatever you want on your plate, but stopping there. No seconds of anything—ever. Once you've done that for a week or so, you'll find that you didn't need seconds after all. In fact, you won't even think about them. It's easier than you think!

5. Individual Servings

Serving dishes look great and remind us of warm family get-togethers, but they make it oh so easy to keep going back for "one more bite." If you are struggling to stick to the "one and done" rule, try taking the willpower out of the equation: Make sure there are no seconds to go back for! One serving for everybody. If they (or you) want more, let 'em grab a bag of baby carrots. If they don't want the baby carrots, they weren't still hungry after all.

6. Divide and Conquer

Remember how you don't feel completely full until fifteen minutes after you stop eating? Make this work for you by having a healthy low-calorie first part to your meal. The salad course is an easy way to do this. Having a salad (easy on the dressing) ahead of your meal not only gives you your full quota of vitamins but also ensures that by the time the high-calorie meats, sauces, and starches come along, you're already half full and not feeling such an urgent need to eat. Overall, you end up eating fewer calories and having a more enjoyable meal. Soups are another great way to blunt your appetite and make dinner more elegant.

Good Fat

Remember when *fat* was a naughty word? When it was the cause of obesity, heart disease, cancer, diabetes, and pretty much any evil we could think of?

My, how times have changed. Thanks in part to better dietary science and in part to Dr. Atkins's revolution, we now accept fat as an essential part of good health. It forms our cell membranes, keeps our skin supple, and builds our brain. It can reduce cholesterol and prevent heart disease. It can even help us lose weight.

Not just any fat, however. The good fats are the *unsaturated* ones: the vegetable, nut, and fish oils. We want to get more of these in our diets. Fats that are solid at body temperature—beef, pork, chicken, and dairy—will solidify in us, too. There, these *saturated* fats really do cause cardiovascular disease—heart attacks and strokes. Picture a pan of bacon fat congealing into a solid white mass; that's what happens in your arteries, too.

Even worse than saturated fats are *trans*fats, which are liquid fats that are made solid through a manufacturing process. Why would anyone want to do that to a perfectly decent vegetable oil? To make margarine, originally, which was created as a

TRANSFAT ALERT

Beware of wolves wearing sheep's clothing, and of saturated fats disguised as unsaturated fats. You won't find transfats on any ingredients list. That's because they are a category of fat and can come in many guises. The most common types of transfat in packaged foods are hydrogenated and partially hydrogenated oils. When you see these on an ingredients list, think transfat. *Think* danger. *Most common sources: margarines, vegetable shortening, packaged cookies, crackers, desserts, and chips. Anything baked or fried with oil and meant to stay on the supermarket shelf for a long time is a likely culprit.*

The other big source of transfats is fast-food french fries (and onion rings). Fast-food companies use hydrogenated oil in their deep-fat fryers because it doesn't go rancid as quickly as plain vegetable oil. (Back when they used beef fat to fry french fries, it was actually slightly better for your heart. Tasted better, too.)

Now that transfats have been recognized as a major contributor to cardiovascular disease, companies are required to list them on their nutrition labels. Look for transfat listed below saturated fat. If it says 0, you're safe. Because this is now a requirement, more and more companies are switching away from transfats, so keep checking those packages on your favorite foods. There are now plenty of margarine spreads, crackers, and other foods that are transfat-free.

cheaper substitute for butter. Unfortunately, turning these liquid vegetable oils solid made them clog arteries and raise bad cholesterol levels even more than butter.

Because solid fats (saturated and trans) are more stable than liquid fats, they take longer to break down and turn rancid. Companies love using transfats in their products to extend shelf life. That's why cookies, crackers, and chips can sit on shelves for months and still be good. But it isn't natural, and we, the consumers, end up paying the price.

The solution to the dangers of saturated fat is not to eat less fat but to switch to unsaturated fat. It gets transformed by the body into a good kind of cholesterol, which acts like a Roto-Rooter in our arteries, sweeping them clear of obstructions so blood can flow smoothly. It also tastes great—an important consideration, since fat gives food body and flavor.

Back in the low-fat craze, when people tried to reduce all kinds of fat in their diets and eat more carbohydrates instead as a way both to lose weight and get healthy, rates of cardiovascular disease and obesity got *worse*. Partly, this was because they were cutting good fat as well as bad. Partly, it was because eating a lot of carbohydrates spikes blood-sugar and insulin levels, which tends to make us hungrier, so we eat more calories overall. We become addicted to eating. Eating carbs instead of saturated fat is not the way to go.

On the other hand, people who replace just one hundred calories per day of saturated fat—about a tablespoon of butter—with one hundred calories of unsaturated fat cut their risk of heart attack in *half!* That's right: All you have to do is start dipping your bread in olive oil instead of using butter and your chances of heart attack plummet. That's pretty dramatic, and it comes without any reduction in overall calorie consumption or food enjoyment, because sources of unsaturated fat include some of the tastiest ingredients known to mankind: foods like avocados, cashews, olive oil, sesame seeds, and salmon.

The weight-loss potential from eating fat comes because it tends to make you feel

A FIELD GUIDE TO FAT

Good Fats	Neutral Fats	Bad Fats	Worst Fats
Olive oil	Corn oil	Butter	Hydrogenated oil
Canola oil	Soybean oil	Cheese	Partially
Nuts	Sunflower oil	Whole-fat dairy	hydrogenated oil
Seeds	Poultry	Beef	
Avocados	Chocolate	Pork	
Fish	Coconut	Lamb	

full fast. Remember how your small intestine is responsible for sending those primary "full" signals to the brain? Well, the food that triggers the strongest full signals is fat! Fat is also absorbed into the bloodstream more slowly than carbohydrates or protein, meaning it keeps you full longer. You don't snack as much.

Because unsaturated fats are so good for both your waistline and your arteries, they are one of the stars of my eating program—as they are in the South Beach diet, the Zone, and many others. Not only will they add years to your life; they'll add pleasure, too. As you begin incorporating healthy fats into your diet this week, you'll be eating some of the most scrumptious foods imaginable. These fats will also help you in your goal this week of portion control, because they allow you to feel full on smaller servings. Eat well, in moderation, and guilt-free!

Strategies for Eating More Good Fat

- Use olive oil instead of butter or margarine.
- Fry foods in canola oil instead of butter or margarine.
- Choose olive oil–based salad dressings.
- Snack on cashews, almonds, walnuts, or pecans.
- Sprinkle sunflower seeds on salads.
- Use guacamole as an appetizer and as a substitute for sour cream.
- Add avocado to your sandwiches.
- Eat multigrain bread with lots of nuts and seeds in it.
- Eat natural peanut butter.
- Use sesame seeds and tahini (ground sesame paste) in your cooking.
- Eat darker-fleshed fishes (salmon, trout, mackerel, herring, sardines, tuna, and bluefish).

HEALTH FLASH

There are more reasons to use extra-virgin olive oil than just the fact that it tastes great. "Extra-virgin" means that the oil is the first cold pressing of the olives, done by hand. After that, more oil is extracted from the same olives by the use of machines and solvents. Ironically, this oil is labeled "pure," yet it isn't as pure a product as extra-virgin and can contain chemical residues.

The Portion-Control Habit Date_____

Mission: Perfect Portions

How big is a serving size, anyway? It's actually a lot smaller than most people think! Look at the box on page 94, and then try to make everything you eat today fit those portion sizes. Today's recipe suggestions, extra-filling due to the good fat from olive oil and nuts, are a great place to start.

Mission Accomplished? _____

WALK BOX

HOW FAR? _____

STRENGTH TRAINING? _____

HOW'D IT GO? _____

FOOD FOCUS: PESTO

SUGGESTED RECIPES

Turkey Pesto Wrap (p. 195)

Linguine with Pesto (p. 210)

BREAKFAST_____ LUNCH_____

_____ _____

DINNER_____ SNACKS_____

_____ _____

DRINKS_____ DESSERTS_____

_____ _____

WATER

1 2 3 4 5 6 7 8

NOTES

_____

_____

_____

_____

_____

_____

_____

_____

_____

_____

_____

_____

The Portion-Control Habit   Date_____

Mission: Smaller Dishes

Contain that habit! This week, readjust your inner concept of what a serving size is. What better way to start than by shrinking your bowls and plates? We tend to fill up whatever dish holds our meal, whether it's a cereal bowl or a dinner plate. Starting today, use smaller dishes to trick your mind into eating less. If you don't have smaller dishes, go ahead and buy some. The investment will pay you back many times over.

Mission Accomplished? _____

WALK BOX

HOW FAR? _____

STRENGTH TRAINING? _____

HOW'D IT GO? _____

FOOD FOCUS: NUTS

SUGGESTED RECIPES

Cashew Chicken Stir-Fry (p. 220)

Lemon Almond Cookies (p. 240)

BREAKFAST_____ LUNCH_____

_____ _____

DINNER_____ SNACKS_____

_____ _____

DRINKS_____ DESSERTS_____

_____ _____

WATER ①②③④⑤⑥⑦⑧

NOTES

_____

_____

_____

_____

_____

_____

_____

_____

_____

_____

_____

_____

_____

_____

The Portion-Control Habit

WEEK 3   WEDNESDAY

Mission: Skinny Glasses

How did the smaller dishes work for you yesterday? Isn't it amazing how a change so obvious can make such a difference? Use them again today, but now change your glassware, too. Get rid of any wide glasses you have. Wide glasses lead to wide people! We tend to drink much more from wide glasses than from narrow ones, so select glasses that reflect your vision of how you want to look: long and slender!

Mission Accomplished? _____

WALK BOX

HOW FAR? _____

STRENGTH TRAINING? _____

HOW'D IT GO? _____

FOOD FOCUS: OLIVE OIL

SUGGESTED RECIPES

Bow-Tie Pasta with Broccoli Rabe (p. 211)

South of France Chicken Salad (p. 204)

BREAKFAST_____ LUNCH_____

_____ _____

DINNER_____ SNACKS_____

_____ _____

DRINKS_____ DESSERTS_____

_____ _____

WATER 1 2 3 4 5 6 7 8

NOTES

_____

_____

_____

_____

_____

_____

_____

_____

_____

_____

_____

_____

The Portion-Control Habit

WEEK 3   THURSDAY

Mission: One and Done

For many of us, surplus calories don't come with our first helping of food, but with all the little extras: seconds, picking at the roasting pan, finishing off the kids' leftovers, and so on. A scoop here, a bite there—it all adds up to hundreds of unnecessary calories. Today, break that habit. You get one plate of food at mealtimes; when it's gone, you're done. Get your belly to fully accept that idea, internalize it as a habit, and watch the pounds melt away.

Mission Accomplished? _____

WALK BOX

HOW FAR? _____

STRENGTH TRAINING? _____

HOW'D IT GO? _____

FOOD FOCUS: NATURAL PEANUT BUTTER

SUGGESTED RECIPES

New PB&J Sandwich (p. 196)

Spicy Peanut Noodles (p. 214)

BREAKFAST_____   LUNCH_____

_____   _____

DINNER_____   SNACKS_____

_____   _____

DRINKS_____   DESSERTS_____

_____   _____

WATER   1   2   3   4   5   6   7   8

NOTES

_____

_____

_____

_____

_____

_____

_____

_____

_____

_____

_____

_____

The Portion-Control Habit

WEEK 3   FRIDAY

Mission: Individual Servings

Were you able to stick to the one-plate-per-meal rule? Here's another tip for achieving the same thing: Plan your single serving in advance. Figure out how much of each food is a serving and parcel it out; then put any leftovers away *before* you start eating. Your brain is much better at controlling what you consume when it isn't getting "yahoo" signals from your taste buds. Do this between meals, too: A drink serving is eight ounces, even if it comes in twenty-ounce bottles! Don't drink from the twenty-ouncer, because you know you'll keep going.

Mission Accomplished? _____

WALK BOX

HOW FAR? _____

STRENGTH TRAINING? _____

HOW'D IT GO? _____

FOOD FOCUS: AVOCADOS

SUGGESTED RECIPES

Tuna and Radish Salad with Creamy Avocado Dressing (p. 199)

Black Bean and Avocado Chili (p. 208)

BREAKFAST_____ LUNCH_____

_____ _____

DINNER_____ SNACKS_____

_____ _____

DRINKS_____ DESSERTS_____

_____ _____

WATER 1 2 3 4 5 6 7 8

NOTES

_____

_____

_____

_____

_____

_____

_____

_____

_____

_____

_____

_____

The Portion-Control Habit   Date_____

WEEK 3   SATURDAY

Mission: Divide and Conquer

Today, conquer your appetite by dividing it up. To prevent that unstoppable "Gotta eat" urge from steamrolling you, start your dinner with a course designed to blunt your appetite. Any soup or salad will do. Raw vegetables with a healthy dip would be another great idea. Whatever it is, remember to reduce the size of the entrée accordingly—because we all know we'll eat pretty much whatever's put in front of us!

Mission Accomplished? _____

WALK BOX

HOW FAR? _____

STRENGTH TRAINING? _____

HOW'D IT GO? _____

FOOD FOCUS: FIRST COURSES

SUGGESTED RECIPES

Rainbow Pepper Medley (p. 228)

Chicken, Pear, Pecan, and Blue Cheese Salad (p. 202)

BREAKFAST_____ LUNCH_____

_____ _____

DINNER_____ SNACKS_____

_____ _____

DRINKS_____ DESSERTS_____

_____ _____

WATER 1 2 3 4 5 6 7 8

NOTES

_____

_____

_____

_____

_____

_____

_____

_____

_____

_____

_____

_____

_____

The Portion-Control Habit   Date_____

WEEK 3   SUNDAY WRAP-UP

THE PERFECT SUPPORT SYSTEM

PLANNING
Three smart behaviors I can adopt next week to support my eating goals:

1. _____

2. _____

3. _____

EDUCATION
What I've learned so far:

NEW HABITS	FOOD SOLUTIONS
Intentional Eating	Water
Breakfast	Whole Grains and Legumes
Portion Control	Good Fat

REPETITION
This week's behaviors:

(Put a ✓ next to those you'll keep doing, an X next to those that weren't useful to you, and an ➤ next to those that you'll try again later.)

1. ___ Realistic Portions   4. ___ One and Done

2. ___ Smaller Dishes   5. ___ Individual Servings

3. ___ Skinny Glasses   6. ___ Divide and Conquer

Other Portion-Control Habits you thought of this week:

_____

_____

Four behaviors from the past three weeks that are becoming habits:

1. _____

2. _____

3. _____

4. _____

FLEXIBILITY

Three ways I can make these habits work better for me:

1. _____
2. _____
3. _____

EXERCISE

Miles/steps walked this week: _____

_____

Other exercise: _____

_____

_____

CELEBRATION!

Three things I'm grateful for this week:

1. _____
2. _____
3. _____

TRANSFORMATION

I surprised myself this week by: _____

NOTES

_____

_____

_____

_____

_____

_____

_____

10. Week 4
The Slow-Food Habit

After three weeks of terrific diet changes, it's time to slowwwwwww things down with the slow-food habit. What on earth is slow food? you ask. It's exactly the opposite of fast food! The Slow Food movement, which started in Italy, began as a reaction to the way fast food malnourishes us and corrupts traditional mealtimes. It's a call to return to a time when food was appreciated for its natural goodness.

Fast food is aptly named, because a lot of our attraction to it has to do with time. It requires no effort on our part, and it shows up two minutes after we ask for it. But this convenience becomes very inconvenient when it results in disease, weight gain, and a reduced quality of life.

There are a number of ways you might incorporate the slow-food habit into your own life. If you have the time to cook traditional meals and eat them with your family, that can be a blessing for both your health and your family dynamics. A lot of sharing of the day's events happens at the dinner table and might not happen otherwise. Meal habits can set the tone for many other parts of life, as well. The family that rushes through meals, or shovels something down in the car on the way to other engagements, tends to be stressed out in other areas of life, too. Which came first, the chicken or the egg? A time crunch between work and play can lead to meals being sacrificed. But the family that manages to maintain the sacredness of the dinner hour carries this relaxed attitude into other activities, as well. The emphasis is on doing one thing at a time, doing it right, and enjoying it thoroughly, rather than squeezing in as much as possible.

More and more research shows that the closer foods are to their natural state— the less processed they are—the better they are for you. We don't need processed food, because we already have a fantastic food processor of our own—the body. What do you think those teeth and that stomach are for? Not for instant rice, I can tell you that. Your body works best when it gets food that takes awhile to break down. It likes food that is *slowly* broken down, because that's what it is designed for. When you eat the simple carbohydrates in junk food and fast food, they instantly enter the bloodstream; that's like putting jet fuel in your car. It burns too hot, too fast, and destroys the engine.

Slow food is food that produces a slow, steady burn in your system. Just because it is slow to digest, however, doesn't mean it needs to be slow to prep and cook. Many vegetables are fast to cook but slow to digest (or are good raw, which makes them even slower to digest). The recipes in this book use natural foods and easy cooking techniques to deliver delectable meals with lots of health benefits in less than thirty minutes. With a little advance planning and a few simple tricks, you can keep your prep time under control and still turn out beautiful meals most nights without having to resort to a box, jar, or frozen entrée.

The supermarket is a very different place from the way it was ten years ago. Food companies have come up with lots of ways of doing the prep work for us. The one you're probably already familiar with is prewashed salad greens in bags. I have no problem with these, because I believe they make people eat more salad. Sure,

I don't want companies to do the work of digesting my food for me, but if they want to take care of the washing, peeling, and chopping, fantastic.

washing and spinning greens isn't that big a deal, but it's just enough to make us consider skipping the greens. Being able to rip open a bag and have a salad instantly removes all the resistance. A salad a day will certainly keep the doctor away—and save you more in medical bills than you'd save by buying heads of lettuce and washing them.

That's just one example of the mind-set I'll help you foster this week—thinking about ways to stock your refrigerator with easy vegetable solutions. I don't want companies to do the work of *digesting* my food for me, but if they want to take care of the washing, peeling, and chopping, fantastic. The days of mushy cans of peas are gone. We've made a lot of progress in ways to freeze foods so that they stay delicious and retain their nutrients. You could argue that there are some fringe benefits to buying your broccoli fresh and doing the prep work yourself. You burn a few calories washing and chopping. It connects you more directly with the food supply and with the past. And I think there's something meditative and pleasant about working with fresh whole foods. Still, I can make an excellent case for the beauty of broccoli florets that are ready to dump into the stir-fry pan. They are just as healthy, and so easy that they take away whatever allure fast food might have. It all depends on what works for you.

Slow food means different things to different people. That's where the flexibility of my plan comes in handy. Make a committed effort this week to consider my slow-food suggestions, throw out the ones that don't apply, and find the two or three that really add satisfaction to your life. Maybe slowing down mealtimes will be just the ticket to changing your relationship with food. Maybe that can't happen in your current life, but learning shortcuts to getting more veggies into you that can be slowly digested will be a lifesaver. There is no right or wrong pick, so long as you keep the ultimate goal in mind: a lifetime of healthy, delicious, and pleasurable eating.

SIX STRATEGIES FOR DEVELOPING YOUR SLOW-FOOD HABIT

1. GO INTERNATIONAL

In America, people developed eating traditions that have generally revolved around a big hunk of protein in the middle of the plate, with little bits of vegetables and potatoes on the sides. This is partly because of our frontier past. Fresh vegetables were hard to come by, but beef was wandering around everywhere!

When you encourage people to eat more vegetables, they think it means sticking with this classic approach but changing the ratios: small meat, big veggies. This doesn't sound very exciting, because vegetables on their own can be . . . well, boring.

People in other cultures, especially Asian ones, have a different solution. They take the small bits of meat, combine them with lots of vegetables, cook it all together, and pour some delicious sauce over the top. The meat and sauce contribute the flavor, the vegetables add crunch and vitamins, and—*presto*—you've got a delicious, healthy, and affordable meal with no boring bites!

Stir-fries are just one example of different ways to start thinking about dinner. Hearty one-pot soups and stews are another. India's cuisine is particularly heavy on the vegetables—and much easier to cook than people think. Take Morocco's couscous, France's ratatouille, Mexico's burritos and enchiladas; almost every culture has come up with brilliant ways to make vegetables yummy. Start experimenting with this week's recipes and watch your family perk up at the dinner table.

2. Eat in Courses

The cultures of the Mediterranean got a three-thousand-year head start on us in perfecting the mealtime experience, so we might have a thing or two to learn from them. One thing you'll notice in Greece, Italy, France, or Spain is that rather than dumping everything on the table, American-style, a series of small courses comes out gradually. In Italy, for example, you might start off with artichokes or an antipasto of tomatoes, basil, and fresh mozzarella, followed by a pasta or soup, then by a meat or fish dish, and then by dessert and espresso. You have only one or two things to focus on at once, allowing you to savor each flavor and to enjoy the anticipation of knowing something different is coming next. It's a good way of training yourself to crave quality instead of quantity in your food. It's also a good way of getting in your vegetables *first*; I'll give you some excellent recipes for turning veggies into snazzy hors d'oeuvres and finger foods.

If having four courses doesn't exactly sound like a weight-loss plan to you, that's because you're thinking in American-size portions. The meat serving would look very small by our standards—certainly not enough to fill you up, but that's the point. It doesn't have to. It's just one player in the symphony. Gradual eating of many different foods is an excellent way to make sure you get a wide variety of vitamins and nutrients without overeating. As I mentioned in chapter 7, "The Intentional Eating Habit," spacing your eating out lets your sense of fullness catch up with you before it's too late!

Eating several courses does take a long time. Italians will linger over dinner for two or three hours. Obviously, we can't do that most nights. The pace of modern life won't allow it. But do try it at least once a week. The relaxed conversation among family and friends that happens as a slow-food dinner rolls along is as nice a way to pass an evening as there is. Why rush through dinner so you can go see a forgettable movie instead?

3. Plan Ahead

These days, not many of us have two hours to prepare dinner—or even one!—so the biggest key to enjoying slow food is to plan ahead. Making one lasagne takes some time; making two takes virtually no extra time, so make two, pop that second one in the freezer, and take it out when you need it.

Many an intention to use brown rice has been scuttled by the sudden discovery, half an hour before dinner, that it takes forty-five minutes to cook! Of course, most of that time doesn't require your involvement at all. Your role takes about a minute: pot, water, rice, salt, flame. That makes brown rice a great high-nutrition, low-effort food, so an hour before dinner, just remember to tell yourself, *Start the rice*. A roast chicken is another healthy and satisfying food that takes very little effort to cook—as long as you remember to get it in the oven two hours ahead of time.

The roast vegetables in Autumn Harvest Medley (p. 229) take an hour in the oven, but they are equally good the day after, so make them in the evening, while you're doing other things, and just microwave them the next day.

4. Share

Nobody makes serious food for just themselves. Eating is a communal act. Having other people around is what turns sustenance into pleasure. If you have a whole family that you cook for, you already have incentive to create a wholesome meal. If you don't, invite some friends over to help you celebrate your foray into slow food.

5. Soup's On

Soup is genius. What better way to make vegetables and whole grains delicious than to slowly cook them in a salty, savory broth? Soup's easy to make, versatile, and, best of all, *the whole thing tastes better the next day*! And even better the day after that! That means several meals of good food with minimal work.

Soup is also low-density food. That's a big appeal of slow-food cooking. Unlike fast food, where it only takes a few bites of meat, cheese, and fried potatoes to wolf down half a day's calories, soup can be eaten only one spoonful at a time. Plus, a lot of soup is water (except for very creamy soups, which you should stay away from). Water has no calories. By the time you finish a bowl of soup, you've been eating for a while, have probably gotten a lot of vitamins, and have blunted your appetite without consuming a massive amount of calories. You'll find it much easier to eat a modest main course and not feel hungry.

Soup can also be a main course. Again, it's a way of changing the ratio of veggies to meat while still being supremely satisfied with the result. Try some soup recipes this week and discover a whole world beyond Campbell's.

6. Embrace the Package

I'm no fanatic. I want you to eat more natural foods, and I don't care what shortcuts you take to get there. Prewashed salad greens, canned black or kidney beans, frozen vegetables, even precooked salmon and shrimp cocktail from the deli—it's all good. I'm not concerned with you developing character through hard work. I'm concerned with you developing good eating habits, whatever the route. If you know of ways to skip the work and still get the benefits, go for it. What you need to avoid is not packaged food but *processed* food, and it's easy to tell the difference. Just glance at the ingredients. If there are things there you don't recognize, things you wouldn't find growing, walking, or swimming in the world, then probably the food isn't very good for you. But a frozen package of blueberries? Yum!

Vegetables

Few things are as pretty as a bowl piled with vegetables of every color: the deep red of a ripe tomato; the vibrant green of spinach or broccoli rabe; the yellows and oranges of peppers, carrots, and squash. If we have a natural attraction to these colors, it's because we were meant to eat a variety of such vegetables. As scientists have confirmed over the past ten years, the colors themselves are created by micronutrients in the vegetables, and these micronutrients are essential to our health. Our hunter-gatherer ancestors probably ate a wide variety of plants as they came across them, and their bodies used the substances in these plants to fight disease. Plants were the original medicine, and nothing has changed. It worked for our ancestors, and it can work for us.

The power of fruits and vegetables to keep us healthy is astonishing. Some of the results of a diet high in these natural disease fighters include:

- Weight loss
- Lower blood pressure and lower cholesterol levels
- Reduced risk of heart disease and stroke
- Reduced risk of diabetes
- Reduced risk of cancer
- Fewer intestinal problems
- Fewer incidences of Alzheimer's disease
- Reduced risk of eye disease

For a while, people dreamed of extracting the medicinal substances in vegetables and turning them into the next round of pills. Eating lots of carrots was associated with protection from various cancers, and scientists knew that beta-carotene was one of the substances responsible, so soon they began giving people beta-carotene pills instead of carrots. And you know what happened? It didn't work. The people taking high levels of beta-carotene actually wound up with *higher* rates of cancer than those in the control group.

We don't know exactly why vegetables deliver so much better health than extract pills, but we can make some good guesses. Fruits and vegetables all have hundreds of active compounds in them, only a few of which have been identified in terms of their healing potential. We know beta-carotene has some health benefits, but there are many other carotenoids in carrots, so if you take beta-carotene pills, you miss out on all the others. We may not yet have identified the most potent carotenoids of all, but we know they're in those carrots and tomatoes and squashes!

The ratio of these healing compounds may also be important. Many of them work in sync in the body, repairing cells and defending them from free-radical damage, and they might not be able to do their thing without their cousins on hand. The natural combinations of vitamins, antioxidants, minerals, and other substances in fruits and vegetables may be essential if you want the full benefit of the "health cocktail."

One clear advantage of fruits and vegetables over supplements is that certain substances are missing from the pills. Supplements have no water, fiber, taste, or crunch in them. You already know why water is essential to good health. As I explained earlier, fiber is nearly as important. It's what holds the cell walls of plants together. It can't be broken down by normal digestion, which is a good thing. Instead, it passes through you unchanged, but on the way it binds with cholesterol and carries it out. This means less cholesterol is around to cause blockages in your arteries.

Part of the benefit of a diet high in fruits and vegetables comes simply because if you are eating more of them, you're eating less of something else, and usually that something else is meat. Meat packs a lot of calories into a fairly small package, meaning you're more likely to eat extra calories. Vegetables are low in calories and take awhile to chew, slowing you down and making you eat less (but feel full because of the fiber). And among dietary substances, meat, high in saturated fat and other unhealthy chemicals, is the biggest cause of heart disease and cancer. Low-carb diets like South Beach have you eat more veggies at the expense of refined carbohydrates, with similar health benefits.

Overall, upping your fruit and veggie intake can probably reduce your risk of cancer by 30 percent, stroke by 30 percent, and heart disease by 15 percent. That's a pretty nice package, as I hope you'll discover in this week's recipes (if you haven't already). All the best textures, flavors, and excitement in food come from that rainbow of goodness waiting for you in the garden.

STRATEGIES FOR EATING MORE VEGETABLES

- When you get a sub or sandwich from a deli, ask for extra vegetables.
- Eat salad *before* your main course; if you save it for after, you might not want it.
- Don't drink your veggies. V-8 juice is a fine drink, but it's no substitute for actual vegetables, and it has little fiber.
- Make raw vegetables your main snack food.
- Shrink your steak and bolster your broccoli. Don't skip the steak entirely; take small bites of it for flavor, but fill up on the greens.

THE COLOR OF HEALTH

The pigments nature uses to color various fruits and vegetables come from natural plant chemicals, each of which has certain disease-fighting specialties, as shown on the chart below. Because there is a lot of overlap, with some chemicals showing up in several different colors, and because scientists are learning more and still perfecting their knowledge, it makes more sense to eat a range of vegetables and fruits in all the colors than to concentrate on one group. Still, if you are concerned about a particular disease, you can eat extra vegetables and fruits of whatever color is known to fight it. (And don't forget that these specialized chemicals are in addition to the healthy vitamins and fiber found in all fruits and vegetables.)

Color	Found In	Helps Prevent
Red (lycopene)	Tomatoes Watermelon	Prostate cancer, lung cancer, and stomach cancer
Purple (flavonoids)	Red grapes Red wine Blueberries Eggplant Red cabbage Red peppers Cocoa beans Coffee Beets Plums Apples Strawberries	Heart disease and stroke
Green (lutein and zeaxanthin)	Spinach Collards Arugula	Cataracts, macular degeneration, stomach cancer, colon cancer, and heart disease
Yellow-Green (indole)	Broccoli Cabbage Kale Brussels sprouts	Colon cancer, bladder cancer, and heart disease
Orange (carotene)	Carrots Sweet potatoes Yellow squash Mangoes Cantaloupe	Breast cancer, stomach cancer, mouth and throat cancer, and lung cancer
White (allicin)	Onions Garlic Leeks	Stomach cancer and high cholesterol

- Try veggie burgers. They're really much better than you think. (And this is from a lifelong carnivore!) With enough catsup, mustard, tomato, onion, and lettuce on there, you won't notice anyway.
- Not crazy about the taste of vegetables? Do what the Italians do—liven them up with olive oil, garlic, salt, and maybe a little crushed red pepper.
- Use packaged salad greens and precut vegetables that are ready to go and eat them raw, steamed, or stir-fried. (See Appendix A, "Ten Food Developments That Will Improve Your Life," for some ideas.)
- Eat at restaurants offering exciting vegetarian entrées and salads.
- Make veggie-rich soups.
- Begin dinner with a first course of veggie-based hors d'oeuvres or spreads. See the recipe suggestions to get started.

HEALTH FLASH

You've heard of antioxidants, the micronutrients that prevent heart disease, stroke, cancer, Alzheimer's, and a host of other diseases, but do you know what the most intense source of antioxidants is? It's chocolate, believe it or not. But not just any chocolate; it must be dark chocolate, the darker the better. A serving of dark chocolate has more antioxidants than any fruit or vegetable, more than making up for its high calorie content. In several studies, volunteers who ate dark chocolate experienced drops in blood pressure and cholesterol, and were less likely to develop heart disease. That's why you owe it to your body to treat yourself to occasional snacks of dark chocolate. Think you can handle that?

The Slow-Food Habit   Date_____

WEEK 4   MONDAY

Mission: Go International

Even if you don't know a wok from a chopstick, you can make delicious stir-fries at home with simple ingredients and no fancy equipment. Thai, Indian, and Mexican cooking are equally easy. Tonight, try one of today's suggested recipes, or anything else that tickles your taste buds and gets you out of the old routine.

Mission Accomplished? _____

WALK BOX

HOW FAR? _____

STRENGTH TRAINING? _____

HOW'D IT GO? _____

FOOD FOCUS: INTERNATIONAL CUISINE

SUGGESTED RECIPES

Chicken Mole (p. 221)

Beef and Snow Pea Stir-Fry (p. 224)

BREAKFAST_____ LUNCH_____
_____ _____

DINNER_____ SNACKS_____
_____ _____

DRINKS_____ DESSERTS_____
_____ _____

WATER 1 2 3 4 5 6 7 8

NOTES

_____
_____
_____
_____
_____
_____
_____
_____
_____
_____
_____
_____

The Slow-Food Habit   Date_____

WEEK 4   TUESDAY

Mission: Eat in Courses

Poor you. Your mission for the day is to pamper yourself and your family or friends with a delicious first course before your entrée. The catch? It has to be something healthy. No crackers and cheese! I suggest trying one of the vegetable dishes recommended below. You'll quickly stop thinking about vegetables as the thing you choke down with your meat! Feel free to eat dessert for course three—just be certain to shrink your main course enough that all three courses together could fit on one medium plate comfortably. Now, that's living well!

Mission Accomplished? _____

WALK BOX

HOW FAR? _____

STRENGTH TRAINING? _____

HOW'D IT GO? _____

FOOD FOCUS: VEGETABLE APPETIZERS

SUGGESTED RECIPES

Wilted Spinach Salad with Bacon (p. 200)

Asparagus Van Gogh (p. 226)

BREAKFAST_____ LUNCH_____

_____ _____

DINNER_____ SNACKS_____

_____ _____

DRINKS_____ DESSERTS_____

_____ _____

WATER 1 2 3 4 5 6 7 8

NOTES

_____

_____

_____

_____

_____

_____

_____

_____

_____

_____

_____

_____

_____

The Slow-Food Habit   Date_____

Mission: Plan Ahead

Simple steps like marinating your meat ahead of time can make a huge difference in flavor and tenderness. You'll be amazed how much better things taste with a little advance attention. You'll also be amazed how little of your time is actually involved. Sure, you've got to start thinking the night before (or at least a few hours before), but it takes only a few minutes to get the marinade going, and then you've got more than enough time available for a good walk! Another way to plan ahead is by making enough for two meals; spinach lasagne is a great way to do just that. You'll find many other nourishing slow-cooked meals in this book—how about a stew, simmering on the stove all afternoon until rich, thick, and succulent?

Mission Accomplished? _____

WALK BOX

HOW FAR? _____

STRENGTH TRAINING? _____

HOW'D IT GO? _____

FOOD FOCUS: ADVANCE PLANNING

SUGGESTED RECIPES

Tandoori Chicken Breasts (p. 220)

No-Boil Spinach Lasagne (p. 213)

BREAKFAST_____ LUNCH_____

_____ _____

DINNER_____ SNACKS_____

_____ _____

DRINKS_____ DESSERTS_____

_____ _____

WATER 1 2 3 4 5 6 7 8

NOTES

_____

_____

_____

_____

_____

_____

_____

_____

_____

_____

_____

_____

The Slow-Food Habit   Date_____

WEEK 4   THURSDAY

Mission: Share

Another real rough assignment today. Simply eat a meal with friends or family and eat it around a table, not on a tray. We are far more likely to eat a "real meal," with a variety of foods, if we aren't eating alone. We also tend to eat more slowly, mixing casual conversation in, and that usually means we feel full on fewer calories.

Mission Accomplished? _____

WALK BOX

HOW FAR? _____

STRENGTH TRAINING? _____

HOW'D IT GO? _____

FOOD FOCUS: VEGGIES FIT FOR COMPANY

SUGGESTED RECIPES

Roasted Tomato and Onion Salad (p. 229)

Spinach with Roasted Garlic Cream (p. 231)

BREAKFAST_____ LUNCH_____

_____ _____

DINNER_____ SNACKS_____

_____ _____

DRINKS_____ DESSERTS_____

_____ _____

WATER (1) (2) (3) (4) (5) (6) (7) (8)

NOTES

_____

_____

_____

_____

_____

_____

_____

_____

_____

_____

_____

_____

The Slow-Food Habit   Date_____

WEEK 4   FRIDAY

Mission: Soup's On

The advertising campaign wasn't lying. Soup is good food. It's just a lot more so when you don't get it out of a can! Making soup is easy, almost foolproof, and so healthy. Whether you have it as a lunch, a first course, or a main dish, it's a great way to maximize flavor and vitamins while minimizing calories.

Mission Accomplished? _____

WALK BOX

HOW FAR? _____

STRENGTH TRAINING? _____

HOW'D IT GO? _____

FOOD FOCUS: SOUP

SUGGESTED RECIPES

Apricot Lentil Stew (p. 207)

Smoky Fish Chowder (p. 209)

BREAKFAST_____ LUNCH_____

_____ _____

DINNER_____ SNACKS_____

_____ _____

DRINKS_____ DESSERTS_____

_____ _____

WATER 1 2 3 4 5 6 7 8

NOTES

_____

_____

_____

_____

_____

_____

_____

_____

_____

_____

_____

_____

_____

The Slow-Food Habit   Date_____

WEEK 4   SATURDAY

Mission: Embrace the Package

Do you steer clear of whole foods because you don't want to deal with the washing, the chopping, the cleaning up afterward? If so, then you can still sustain yourself with *wholesome* foods that come ready to cook. Try some today. Take one of the recipe suggestions below, or just explore that aisle of the supermarket and discover some of the healthy new products appearing faster than we can keep track of. See Appendix A, "Ten Food Developments That Will Improve Your Life," for a head start.

Mission Accomplished? _____

WALK BOX

HOW FAR? _____

STRENGTH TRAINING? _____

HOW'D IT GO? _____

FOOD FOCUS: NO-PREP VEGGIES

SUGGESTED RECIPES

Garlicky Cauliflower Mash (p. 230)

Butternut Squash with Tarragon (p. 230)

BREAKFAST_____ LUNCH_____

_____ _____

DINNER_____ SNACKS_____

_____ _____

DRINKS_____ DESSERTS_____

_____ _____

WATER   1   2   3   4   5   6   7   8

NOTES

_____

_____

_____

_____

_____

_____

_____

_____

_____

_____

_____

_____

The Slow-Food Habit   Date_____

THE PERFECT SUPPORT SYSTEM

PLANNING
Three smart behaviors I can adopt next week to support my eating goals:
1. _____
2. _____
3. _____

EDUCATION
What I've learned so far:

NEW HABITS	FOOD SOLUTIONS
Intentional Eating	Water
Breakfast	Whole Grains and Legumes
Portion Control	Good Fat
Slow Food	Vegetables

REPETITION
This week's behaviors:
(Put a ✓ next to those you'll keep doing, an X next to those that weren't useful to you, and an ➤ next to those that you'll try again later.)

1. ___ Go International   4. ___ Share
2. ___ Eat in Courses   5. ___ Soup's On
3. ___ Plan Ahead   6. ___ Embrace the Package

Other Slow-Food Habits you thought of this week:

_____

_____

Six behaviors from the past four weeks that are becoming habits:

1. _____
2. _____
3. _____

4. _____

5. _____

6. _____

FLEXIBILITY

Three ways I can make these habits work better for me:

1. _____
2. _____
3. _____

EXERCISE

Miles/steps walked this week: _____

_____

Other exercise: _____

_____

_____

CELEBRATION!

Three things I'm grateful for this week:

1. _____
2. _____
3. _____

TRANSFORMATION

I surprised myself this week by: _____

NOTES

_____

_____

_____

_____

Do I ever eat for reasons other than hunger?

You bet I do! Eating feels good, even when it's not about survival. Popping something in my mouth for enjoyment now and then simply makes me a card-carrying member of the human race.

Reaching for food can be a way of dealing with discomfort. People have lots of automatic habits they use as a way of comforting themselves. Some bite their nails. Some rub a favorite stone. Some eat.

In a way, eating makes the most sense of the bunch, because eating is the way we were comforted as infants. Back then, if food was going in, we knew everything was okay. We had no other worries! Now, no matter how many worries we have, the sensation of eating is still a shorthand way of telling ourselves that everything is okay.

Things get complicated, however, when eating becomes the exact behavior that leads to weight gain and illness—more worries! But if the reaction to this is to eat for comfort, then a vicious cycle develops. We eat to soothe our anxiety or depression, but the eating fuels more anxiety, causing us to reach for food, which we know we shouldn't be doing . . . and on and on. When your problem and your way of dealing with the problem are the same, you're in trouble.

This is why I feel that compulsive snacking can be a bigger threat to our health than anything we do at mealtimes. Plenty of people out there eat three perfectly sensible meals a day, then "supplement" these calories with a never-ending supply of chips in the office, sodas in the car, and candy on the couch.

By filling out the questionnaire on page 36, you raised your awareness about the reasons why you eat. You learned a thing or two about yourself and have been actively changing your habits. Now you need to ask yourself one important question: Are you a grazer or a traditionalist?

A grazer is someone who does best eating small meals throughout the day. For grazers, the time between meals is too long; they get hungry and become less productive in the hour or two before a meal because all they can do is think about food. Sometimes, this makes them so ravenous that they end up overeating when mealtime finally comes. Even if they manage not to overeat, grazers are bothered by the spikes and drops in blood-sugar levels that come from eating three substantial meals a day with nothing in between. For grazers, the solution is to eat a midmorning and midafternoon snack. This keeps the blood sugar nice and level—in theory, anyway. To be honest, I'm skeptical of grazing. I know it works for some people, and I give you the option of making it a centerpiece of your new diet habits, but I've seen

Are you a grazer or a traditionalist?

more harm than good done in the name of grazing. The problem comes because grazers are supposed to eat smaller meals. All those calories that you consume in your two snacks are supposed to mean you consume fewer calories at mealtime, so your overall calorie intake remains unchanged (or goes down). But snacks are a two-edged sword. If they blunt your appetite at meals, great. Often, however, people eat the snacks, telling themselves how small their dinner will be, but by the time dinner rolls around, they have forgotten all that. The food is on the table, everyone's eating and having fun, so they serve themselves a normal plate of food and eat it. Oops, forgot about that snack three hours ago! Too often, I see people eat three regular meals—with a full day's supply of food energy—plus various snacks, all in the name of health. The result: too many calories over the course of the day and, thus, weight gain.

If you really are a grazer and like to eat small meals, the trick is to make sure your snacks and meals consist of a mix of protein, fat, and carbohydrates, so your energy level stays steady throughout the day. If you are a traditionalist and do best on three square meals a day, this is even more essential.

I'm a traditionalist. I like eating a solid breakfast, lunch, and dinner and not giving food a thought in between. As I said at the beginning of this chapter, there are certainly times when I eat that have nothing to do with hunger, but I try to make them rare. For instance, one habit I've developed is never eating at work. I don't even have to think about it anymore, so it takes no willpower on my part. Work is for work. Home and restaurants are for eating. Sure, somebody is always having a birthday party, complete with cake, in the office. But I never give it a thought. They don't even ask me if I want any anymore.

What's more important, my body has grown accustomed to not eating between meals, so it never desires snacks. Of course, I have to help my body out by giving it enough breakfast and lunch, and the right kinds, so that it has the energy it needs to get through the day.

One reason I prefer the traditional approach is that it makes food less of a centerpiece in my life. When every two hours involves prepping or eating food of some kind, it starts to loom large in your mind. A lot of your self-image can get tied up in your battle against the Food Monster. If you can train your body to eat three times a day and not concern itself with food the rest of the time, you pull the plug on the Food Monster. It starts to lose its power over you.

That's why your first mission during Snack Habit week is *not to snack*. Call it "the nonsnack habit." I'll give you some tips for taking away the temptations that make people snack automatically. You may find that when temptation is removed, you become an entirely different person than you thought you were.

Then again, you may find that without snack breaks, you become a ravenous grump before lunch. If that's the case, you'll want to focus on this week's other tips, which involve ways to deliver high-nutrition jolts in small packages so you can snack your way thin.

Whichever meal plan you set up for yourself, the key is to stick with it and do the same thing every day so that it becomes a habit. When you stop thinking about it and just do it, you know you've succeeded.

Six Strategies for Developing Your Snack Habit

1. Bombproof Your House

How many people do you know who have no real sweet tooth but turn into candy-craving junkies on November 1, knowing that the kids are at school and that bag of Halloween candy waits unprotected in the bedroom? If Halloween doesn't get me, Easter does, as I turn to mush at the sight of marshmallow peeps!

No one manages to curb their snack habit while surrounded by packages of candy, chips, cookies, popcorn, and ice cream, all just begging for a little attention. When you break down and scarf the whole bag of Doritos, or the candy bar you knew perfectly well was "hidden" in the drawer, don't blame willpower. Blame brainpower! Deep down, you knew what was going to happen once you bought those foods, even if you told yourself they were for the kids, or for a special treat. Willpower is something that works best when it isn't tested. That's what you must do for yourself.

If you have junk food in your house, throw it out. Don't feel like you are *wasting* anything. That's a destructive thinking pattern. If you discovered poison in your house and threw it out, you wouldn't think you were wasting it. Well, guess what? That box of doughnuts is poison, the slow-acting kind, and in the long run it'll make you plenty sick.

This one is nonnegotiable. If you are at all serious about getting fit, you have no excuse for bringing junk food into the house to sabotage yourself. Get it out, throw it out, and be amazed at how you can't eat it when it's not around. Then you end up eating an apple or some cashews instead. After a few weeks, when you happen to taste junk food somewhere, you discover an amazing thing: It doesn't taste so good! Once you lose your taste for it, it won't come back.

2. Bombproof Your Office

Clearing the junk food from your house and depositing it in your desk drawer at work or in the glove compartment of your car doesn't count! I know, you can't make everyone else at work stop snacking, and you can't set the vending machines on fire, and you can't stop driving by convenience stores in your car, but there are different levels of temptation. People are much more likely to reach for food if it's within arm's reach, so make your desk a no-food zone. Do the same for your car. The more sanctuaries you have, the less chance the Food Monster has of finding you.

3. Try Tea

What you're really after from a snack may just be something to keep your mouth busy. To find out, try a cup of herbal tea or decaffeinated coffee. Hot drinks like these last a long time, have no calories, and are extremely comforting. By the time you're done sipping them, the Food Monster may have passed you by. Or it may be mealtime already. Remember that spices tend to curb appetite, so try drinks like Indian chai, which are full of exciting flavors to keep you from missing a food snack. Just make sure the drinks themselves aren't caloric.

4. Easy Does It

A submarine sandwich is not a snack! For that matter, you shouldn't follow up a midmorning snack with a full sandwich for lunch. Try dividing that sandwich up and having half for a snack, then half with grapes on the side at lunch. Think the same way about dinner if you have a midafternoon snack: Whatever your snack is, you should very consciously carve that amount of food out of your dinner.

If you snack, it's particularly important to plan your meals in advance. Otherwise, you'll forget you've snacked and end up eating too much. I don't recommend counting calories on a daily basis—too much drudgery—but you might try a spot count on a few of your meals and snacks. Once you get a sense for what, say, three four-hundred-calorie meals plus two two-hundred-calorie snacks should look like, you can just eyeball it after that. Be warned: You may be surprised how small a four-hundred-calorie meal looks.

If you are devoted to dessert, that could serve as one of your snacks. But again, you may be in for a shock: A two-hundred-calorie serving of ice cream is pretty small (but still plenty to satisfy you). The dessert recipes in this book all create servings that contain fewer than two hundred calories. (Both the Guava Granita and the Lemon Almond Cookies are under one hundred!)

5. PROTEIN PERSISTS

If you do decide you are a grazer, make sure your snacks have some protein in them. Protein is more slowly digested than carbohydrates, so you stay full longer, and it doesn't pack the calorie wallop that fat does. Some excellent sources of snack protein are hard-boiled eggs, natural peanut butter, energy bars, yogurt, and nuts. You'll find some yummy suggestions for high-energy snacking in this week's recipe suggestions.

6. FIBER FILLS

Fiber—indigestible material found in fruits, vegetables, beans, and whole grains— is a dieter's best friend. How can something indigestible be good for us? Because fiber takes up space in the stomach and intestines without delivering any calories. It makes us feel full but doesn't make us fat! Not only that, but fiber gets in the way of the carbohydrates in our food and thus it takes longer for the body to digest them, meaning fiber helps control our blood-sugar and insulin levels. Choose fiber in your snacks (fruit is perfect!) and you'll find a little food goes a long way.

Fruit

For many millions of years, the plant kingdom has been developing the perfect food. It's sweet yet healthy, filling yet low in calories, and it comes ready to eat in individual serving sizes. This miracle food is fruit, of course, and it's part of a long-standing agreement between plants and animals: We get the yummy treat in exchange for spreading around the seeds hidden in the fruit. Everybody wins: More seeds get disseminated, which means more fruit for us.

For most of human history, fruit has been a staple of the human diet and probably the primary source of sweetness. That all changed when sugar became cheap and widely available in the seventeenth century. People forgot about the miracle of plucking delicious food straight off the tree and turned toward cakes and cookies instead.

And that's where things went wrong. As people's taste for sweets grew and they consumed more and more desserts and baked goods, obesity and all the diseases that come with it—diabetes, heart disease, cancer, and more—grew, too. Only recently have we finally learned that sweets and fruit are not the same.

It turns out nature was taking care of everyone all along. For while fruits are sweet and delicious, they are also incredibly healthy. Along with the sugars in fruit comes fiber, tough material in the flesh and skins of fruit, which we can't digest. The body has to sort through the fiber and other material to get the sugars, which takes some time, meaning fruit, unlike simple carbs, doesn't spike blood sugar and cause increased insulin production. That fiber also helps to keep your gut running smoothly. And fruits are simply packed with vitamins and micronutrients, meaning they help prevent many diseases, as well as tasting great.

Researchers don't usually separate fruits from vegetables when studying health benefits. They consider them a partnership that works hand in hand to keep you slim, energized, and disease-free. As I mentioned in the previous chapter, you can probably reduce your risk of cancer by 30 percent, stroke by 30 percent, and heart disease by 15 percent by getting five servings a day of fruits and veggies.

With fruit, the question is: When to sneak in those servings? Other than having the occasional fruit salad at brunch, we aren't used to making fruit a part of our meals anymore. Yet fruit goes well with almost everything and makes many other foods taste better. You haven't lived until you've had crisp sliced apples on a turkey sandwich! Since fruit is ready to eat, it also makes the ultimate snack—portable, nutritious, delicious. How many creative ways can you come up with to develop your fruit habit? Use my tips below, and this week's recipe ideas, to get you started.

- Have a grapefruit first thing in the morning. The fiber and vitamin C will get your day off to a superhealthy, high-metabolism, steady-energy start.
- Drink fruit smoothies for breakfast (p. 189).
- Have apples or bananas with natural peanut butter for your snack. That makes an ideal combination of protein, complex carbs, good fat, and lots of vitamins.
- Make all your desserts with fruit, using a minimum of other sugars. An apple crisp with oatmeal crumble never did anybody any harm. Neither did Pears Poached in Wine Sauce (p. 243).
- Replace starchy side dishes, such as french fries or rice, with fruit or fruit salad. Your meal will taste much better, and your pancreas will thank you!
- Don't skimp on fruit. Even if it seems a little pricey in the supermarket, remember that when you buy it, you are buying health. A four-dollar pineapple is a bargain compared to a fat-laden pork chop.
- Keep a bowl filled with a multicolored variety of gorgeous fruit in your kitchen at all times. Having it visible, within reach, and ready to eat makes you much more likely to grab some fruit than if it's buried in the crisper drawer.
- If peeling and prepping keeps you from eating more fruit, don't hesitate to buy the containers of cubed melon, pineapple, mango, and peach. (But stay away from ones that are stored in a sugar syrup.)

NOT ALL FRUITS ARE CREATED EQUAL

Some fruits raise your blood-sugar level more than others. It all depends on how dense their sugar is and how much fiber, nutrients, and other material they have in them. You can compare by looking at a glycemic index—numbers that show how fast a food's carbohydrates are absorbed into the blood compared to white bread, which has a glycemic index of 100. In general, melons and tropical fruits have a higher glycemic index than do citrus fruits, apples and pears, or berries. (But all of these numbers are much lower than those for potatoes, refined grains, and sugar.)

Watermelon	72	Orange	42
Cantaloupe	65	Peach	42
Raisins	64	Strawberries	40
Pineapple	59	Apple	38
Kiwi	53	Pear	38
Banana	52	Grapefruit	25
Mango	51	Cherries	22

The Snack Habit   Date_____

Mission: Bombproof Your House

The secret to weight-loss success is to put less pressure on yourself and more on your environment. Put yourself in a no-fail environment and you won't fail, plain and simple. Today is the day you set up that environment. Make your home a sanctuary from temptation. At some moment when you're feeling strong, go through the cupboards and throw out all the junk food—every bit of it! Do the same for any other room in the house where you might have a hidden stash. And once it's gone, remind yourself of the one cardinal rule: It can never, ever come into your sanctuary again. If you want to break the snack habit, put yourself in a snack-free zone. Make sure there's nothing easy to grab, and fortify yourself with a substantial breakfast and lunch so that you will have everything you need to sail through until dinner.

Mission Accomplished? _____

WALK BOX

HOW FAR? _____

STRENGTH TRAINING? _____

HOW'D IT GO? _____

FOOD FOCUS: LUNCHES WITH STAYING POWER

SUGGESTED RECIPES

Pork Tenderloin Sandwich (p. 196)

Blackened Chicken Salad (p. 203)

BREAKFAST_____ LUNCH_____

_____ _____

DINNER_____ SNACKS_____

_____ _____

DRINKS_____ DESSERTS_____

_____ _____

WATER 1 2 3 4 5 6 7 8

NOTES

_____

_____

_____

_____

_____

_____

_____

_____

_____

_____

_____

_____

_____

The Snack Habit

WEEK 5 TUESDAY

Mission: Bombproof Your Office

Years ago, I made my office a no-food zone. I simply don't eat while I'm working. You'd be amazed how much mental energy this saves me. No more agonizing over whether to have a slice of birthday cake or not; it's not even an option. Starting today, do the same for yourself. Eating while you work is no longer an option—whatever and wherever your work is. Once your body, and everyone around you, knows this, you'll find that the internal and external signals to snack disappear within a week.

Mission Accomplished? _____

WALK BOX

HOW FAR? _____

STRENGTH TRAINING? _____

HOW'D IT GO? _____

FOOD FOCUS: ALTERNATIVES TO JUNK FOOD

SUGGESTED RECIPES

Spicy Tamari Almonds (p. 238)

Cashew-Ginger Trail Mix (p. 238)

BREAKFAST_____ LUNCH_____

_____ _____

DINNER_____ SNACKS_____

_____ _____

DRINKS_____ DESSERTS_____

_____ _____

WATER 1 2 3 4 5 6 7 8

NOTES

_____

_____

_____

_____

_____

_____

_____

_____

_____

_____

_____

_____

_____

The Snack Habit Date_____

WEEK 5 WEDNESDAY

Mission: Try Tea

A lot of snacking is really just about keeping the mouth busy—which is really just about boredom. Sometimes we are going to be faced with boring hours on the job or at home. Today, when your mouth needs some action, try a cup of herbal tea instead. It's delicious, calorie-free, and has a variety of health benefits. It even counts toward your water goal! As do the cold teas in today's suggested recipes.

Mission Accomplished? _____

WALK BOX

HOW FAR? _____

STRENGTH TRAINING? _____

HOW'D IT GO? _____

FOOD FOCUS: TEAS

SUGGESTED RECIPES

Holiday Spice Tea (p. 245)

Peachy Green Tea Punch (p. 245)

BREAKFAST_____ LUNCH_____

_____ _____

DINNER_____ SNACKS_____

_____ _____

DRINKS_____ DESSERTS_____

_____ _____

WATER 1 2 3 4 5 6 7 8

NOTES

_____

_____

_____

_____

_____

_____

_____

_____

_____

_____

_____

_____

_____

The Snack Habit Date_____

WEEK 5   THURSDAY

Mission: Easy Does It

I have mixed feelings about snacking. It's too easy to make it an excuse to eat five meals a day. To see if you do better with a number of small meals throughout the day, plan your lunch and dinner ahead of time; then take a portion of one (or both) of those and make that your snack (or snacks). That way, you'll be sure your total calorie intake doesn't change. If you are a confirmed dessert eater, use that as one of your snacks, and carve that many calories out of your dinner.

Mission Accomplished? _____

WALK BOX

HOW FAR? _____

STRENGTH TRAINING? _____

HOW'D IT GO? _____

FOOD FOCUS: HEALTHY DESSERTS

SUGGESTED RECIPES

Chocolate Fondue with Fresh Fruit (p. 244)

Sugar-Free Apple Pie (p. 242)

BREAKFAST_____ LUNCH_____

_____ _____

DINNER_____ SNACKS_____

_____ _____

DRINKS_____ DESSERTS_____

_____ _____

WATER 1 2 3 4 5 6 7 8

NOTES

_____

_____

_____

_____

_____

_____

_____

_____

_____

_____

_____

_____

The Snack Habit   Date_____

WEEK 5   FRIDAY

Mission: Protein Persists

People get snacks all wrong. When you snack on sweets or bread products, you put yourself on the carbohydrate roller coaster, which can leave you just as hungry as when you started. Today, include some protein in your snack and you'll find that it stays with you a lot longer—all the way to mealtime, in fact. Try a handful of nuts, sliced turkey, an egg, or some of the smart snacks in today's suggested recipes.

Mission Accomplished? _____

WALK BOX

HOW FAR? _____

STRENGTH TRAINING? _____

HOW'D IT GO? _____

FOOD FOCUS: PROTEIN SNACKS

SUGGESTED RECIPES

Prosciutto, Fig, and Melon Salad (p. 202)

Spinach-Feta Bites (p. 237)

BREAKFAST_____ LUNCH_____

_____ _____

DINNER_____ SNACKS_____

_____ _____

DRINKS_____ DESSERTS_____

_____ _____

WATER ⑴ ⑵ ⑶ ⑷ ⑸ ⑹ ⑺ ⑻

NOTES

_____

_____

_____

_____

_____

_____

_____

_____

_____

_____

_____

_____

_____

The Snack Habit   **Date**_____

WEEK 5   SATURDAY

Mission: Fiber Fills

Yesterday, you tried a high-protein snack. Today, add fiber into the mix. Fiber, found in fruits, vegetables, and whole grains, slows down your digestion, so you'll eat smaller amounts but feel full for hours. Since it has zero calories, it's a great weight-loss secret.

Mission Accomplished? _____

WALK BOX

HOW FAR? _____

STRENGTH TRAINING? _____

HOW'D IT GO? _____

FOOD FOCUS: HIGH-FIBER SNACKS

SUGGESTED RECIPES

Roasted Red Pepper Spread (p. 235)

Sugar-Free Pumpkin Pie (p. 243)

BREAKFAST_____ LUNCH_____

_____ _____

DINNER_____ SNACKS_____

_____ _____

DRINKS_____ DESSERTS_____

_____ _____

WATER 1 2 3 4 5 6 7 8

NOTES

_____

_____

_____

_____

_____

_____

_____

_____

_____

_____

_____

_____

_____

The Snack Habit

WEEK 5   SUNDAY WRAP-UP
THE PERFECT SUPPORT SYSTEM

PLANNING

Three smart behaviors I can adopt next week to support my eating goals:

1. _____
2. _____
3. _____

EDUCATION

What I've learned so far:

NEW HABITS	FOOD SOLUTIONS
Intentional Eating	Water
Breakfast	Whole Grains and Legumes
Portion Control	Good Fat
Slow Food	Vegetables
Snack	Fruits

REPETITION

This week's behaviors:

(Put a ✓ next to those you'll keep doing, an X next to those that weren't useful to you, and an ➤ next to those that you'll try again later.)

1. ___ Bombproof Your House   4. ___ Easy Does It
2. ___ Bombproof Your Office   5. ___ Protein Persists
3. ___ Try Tea   6. ___ Fiber Fills

Other Snack Habits you thought of this week:

_____

Eight behaviors from the past five weeks that are becoming habits:

1. _____   5. _____
2. _____   6. _____
3. _____   7. _____
4. _____   8. _____

FLEXIBILITY

Three ways I can make these habits work better for me:

1. _____
2. _____
3. _____

EXERCISE

Miles/steps walked this week: _____
_____

Other exercise: _____
_____
_____

CELEBRATION!

Three things I'm grateful for this week:

1. _____
2. _____
3. _____

TRANSFORMATION

I surprised myself this week by: _____

NOTES

_____
_____
_____
_____
_____
_____
_____

12. Week 6
The Restaurant Habit

Congratulations! You've made it to the last week of the program! By now, you're eating smart breakfasts, you've banned junk food from the house permanently, and you've even gotten your family to discover that they like broccoli more than they ever imagined. Time to close a big loophole.

Learning about nutrition and how to cook healthy meals that taste good is a big step, but it's only part of the smart-eating journey. Too many popular diet books stop there. What I've tried to do in this book is deal with the realities of how we all eat, and the reality is that most of us eat out half the time. Since we tend to indulge a bit more when eating out, meals outside the home actually account for *more* than 50 percent of our calories. Any diet that doesn't deal with this isn't going to have much impact.

Eating out includes sit-down restaurants; fast-food, sandwich, and take-out joints; and all the other places ready to hand us hot food at a moment's notice. It's a reality of our fast-paced lives that we're going to use these places some of the time. And there's nothing wrong with that. I don't want you to eat out less. I just want you to learn some strategies to make restaurants work for you, not against you.

Today's restaurants seem to be moving in two directions at once. On one hand, they're clued in to the fact that a lot of us want healthy choices and will order them if available. More and more restaurants are offering smart entrées. At the same time, restaurants seem to be competing with one another to see who can offer the biggest, saltiest, fattiest, most overwhelming dinner options known to mankind. When Bennigan's offers a Bleu Cheese Filet, the whole country is in trouble. I don't know of anyone who really needs a meal like that. But Bennigan's is just in competition with all the other chains, and if customers didn't like their steaks smothered in blue cheese, restaurants wouldn't be offering it. Offering customers *more* for their money is much easier for chains than offering *better*.

Even if you steer clear of these megameals, they may be doing their damage anyway, because they make more modest dinners seem smaller than they really are. Huge restaurant portions make us eat more than we need, even if we leave plenty on the plate, and they get us accustomed to thinking eat such portions are normal, so we end up serving more at home, too.

So what are we to do? Give up restaurants? Far from it! I *love* eating out, and I'm willing to bet you do, too. That's why you're going to like this last week of the program *a lot*. Your assignment, should you choose to accept it, is to eat out at least three times this week. Pretty tough, huh? But here's the catch. To retrain yourself for a whole new set of restaurant habits, use some of this week's six strategies on the days you dine out. Allow yourself as much flexibility as you need to. I'll still suggest one strategy to try each day, but you almost certainly won't be able to put them all into play, so feel free to match up whichever strategies appeal to you with whichever days you have free for a meal out. It's more important that you develop a couple of restaurant strategies into restaurant habits than that you try out every possibility.

THE FIVE COMMANDMENTS OF DINING OUT

From fast food to the fanciest French restaurant, these basic rules will serve you well.
1. Choose fish or chicken over red meat.
2. Choose grilled over fried.
3. Choose veggies or beans over starches.
4. Choose nonsugared drinks.
5. Split (or skip) dessert.

SIX STRATEGIES FOR DEVELOPING YOUR RESTAURANT HABIT

1. LET THEM DO THE SHUCKING

It's a wonder that we don't eat more shellfish. It's very high in protein, virtually fat-free, and incredibly delicious. If you can think of a food that is both healthier and more scrumptious, call me. Yet the problem with shellfish is the prep. Who wants to shell shrimp, scrub mussels, or chase a lobster across the kitchen? So don't.

That's what restaurants are for. Save your restaurant dollars for the healthy food you love to eat but hate to cook. Don't be tempted by the prime rib when you know that this is one of your best chances to buy health.

You can carry this concept beyond shellfish. Any healthy food that's a pain to cook is the one to order when you're out. Artichokes, anyone? Caesar salad? Sushi? You get the idea.

2. GO SPLITSVILLE

A lot of us have this crazy, outdated notion that waiters consider it rude if we go to a restaurant and don't order a lot of food. The truth is, they really don't care; they all pool their tips these days anyway, so don't worry about the size of your bill. Trust me, they'll think a lot worse of you if you order enough food for three people! Splitting an entrée with another person is sometimes the only sensible solution in this world of portions gone wild.

The best part of entrée splitting (other than the inherent romance in it!) is that it allows you to have a more adventurous meal. You save so many calories by eating only half the entrée that you have plenty of leeway to split an appetizer or two or even a dessert. By doing so, you'll also be re-creating the slow-food experience: several small courses of various tasty morsels, instead of one mammoth steak.

Say your dearly beloved doesn't want to split the seafood with you; he wants his precious roast beef. That's fine; split your meal with *yourself*. Ask for a doggie bag and stick half your food in it as soon as it comes. Then not only do you keep your portion well under control but you also have a delicious no-cook meal ready for the microwave tomorrow! Now *that's* a smart habit.

3. SHRIMPY-SIZE ME

One thing I'm not going to suggest you do is avoid fast-food restaurants. In our hectic lives, every now and then they come in handy. Keep using them; just know how to work them to your own benefit. All fast-food places offer the option of small sandwiches—usually the ones they are advertising for only ninety-nine cents—and then the choices go up to large, grande, supergrande, and so on. The chains make most of their money on the big-ticket items (and especially the sodas), but there's no law against getting the small item.

You don't need to stick with the burger routine anymore, either. All the major chains offer some sort of grilled chicken item, which is much lower in fat because the chicken is grilled over a flame instead of fried in fat. Better still, fast-food chains are finally getting serious about salad. Sure, they offered salads in the old days, but let's just say that their resemblance to fresh food was purely coincidental. Not anymore. For example, Burger King's Fire-Grilled Shrimp Salad comes with the hot shrimp in a separate pouch and fresh lettuce, grape tomatoes, cucumber, onions, and carrots on the cool side. Get that with a bottle of water and you are taking good care of yourself. If you are tempted by the wafting smell of bacon cheeseburgers, remember that you are buying health, not as much as you can eat for five bucks. That's the question you want to ask yourself: How can I get the most health and satisfaction later in my day for five bucks?

4. DON'T GET CARB-FOOLED

As I've said earlier in this book, diets that alert Americans to the dangers of eating too many carbs, such as Atkins and South Beach, do us a lot of favors. Reducing carb consumption is important. Unfortunately, too often the message people take away is "Eat anything you want as long as it's not carbs." Equally unfortunate are restaurant chains that give people exactly what they think they want. Take the Carl's Jr. Low-Carb Breakfast Bowl, a pile of eggs, cheese, sausage, ham, and bacon, without a crumb of toast to be found. The calorie load? A mere nine hundred for breakfast. If you've noticed people who eat Breakfast Bowls getting any thinner, let me know. Watch out for the infamous bunless burgers wrapped in lettuce, too. Yes, you save a few calories on the bun, but don't you think that extra-large slab of beef might make up for it?

This trend isn't limited to fast food, either. Plenty of sit-down restaurants have decided that steak alone isn't good enough. They're adding a generous slab of cheese on top, giving you more saturated fat in one meal than you need in a week.

Also, I'll let you in on a little secret of restaurant cooking. As anyone who has worked in a fancy restaurant can tell you, virtually every sauce and many entrées are "finished" with a big ol' hunk of butter. That's why restaurant food often tastes so good. Boom! Up to two hundred more calories added to your meal without even showing up in the menu description.

Don't take your eyes off the prize by fixing them on the number of carbs in a meal. If you're going to look at one nutrient, look at saturated fat (and its cousin, transfat). More important, look at total calories. But at most sit-down restaurants, you won't find nutritional information, which means you'll have to use your instincts. If a dressing, sauce, cream soup, or entrée tastes a little too good, it probably is!

5. BAN THE BUFFET

Whether it's in a Chinese or Indian restaurant or a place that offers a breakfast buffet or a salad bar, the idea of "all you can eat" is a terrible one. Right away, the focus is on getting the most for your money. Even at a classy brunch, the emphasis is on quantity, not quality. It's very difficult to walk into a place with this understanding and *not* overeat. Who can blame you? You want to try everything but don't want to leave five half-eaten plates of food . . . and then there's that dessert bar waiting at the end.

Under any circumstance, buffets are a bad idea. Cut them out of your life entirely and instead frequent restaurants that emphasize quality and health, not quantity. If you have to go to a buffet for an important family or business event, keep in mind your old "one and done" rule: No matter how much free food surrounds you, you still need only one plateful. If others give you a hard time, ask them why they feel compelled to overeat.

6. Avoid the Bread Bomb

It's so comforting. You plunk down in a nice restaurant and instantly a basket of crusty fresh bread hits your table, still steaming from the oven. With that cute bowl of olive oil next to it, you can't help but eat a slice, or three. Don't do it! That innocent-looking loaf is a good way to turn a decent meal into a calorie train wreck. We generally don't eat less of our meal because we already ate the bread. We paid for that meal and we are darn well gonna force it down! A study of Italian restaurants showed that the average diner ate almost three hundred calories worth of bread and olive oil or butter with a meal. Do that twice a week and it can add up to nearly ten pounds a year! If it helps, ask the waiter to take the bread basket away so you won't be tempted.

If you order something small, like a bowl of soup, then the bread can make sense. But even then, if you eat it with butter, you are getting a nutritionally empty hit of simple carbs and saturated fat. Using the olive oil helps, but skipping the bread altogether is the best solution of all.

Seafood

Back in Week 3, I explained the benefits of unsaturated fat, but I left out the most special kind of all. Omega-3 fat is so good for you that it deserves a category all its own. It's found primarily in fish, as well as in walnuts, canola oil, and flaxseed. Think of omega-3 as a vitamin rather than a fat, because you only need about a gram of it a day—about twice the amount of vitamin C you need. Remember the cod-liver oil your grandparents were forced to eat as children? Turns out it really was good for you, and the reason was the omega-3! It's essential to the function of the brain, the eye, and the reproductive system. It keeps the heart beating on time and reduces inflammation throughout the body, protecting against everything from cardiovascular disease to autoimmune diseases like lupus, rheumatoid arthritis, and Crohn's.

One large study showed that getting just one gram per day of omega-3 cut people's risk of sudden heart attack in half, and had a smaller positive effect on their overall chance of heart disease. But how much does the average American get per day? Just one-tenth of that.

To get your daily gram of omega-3, you can eat one serving of fish, walnuts, or canola oil. Not all fish carry equal amounts of omega-3. The fattier fish have the most. That means northern cold-water fish, such as bluefish, mackerel, salmon, herring, and trout, are excellent sources. Sardines are another excellent source. Tuna and swordfish aren't bad, either.

WHERE CAN I GET MY OMEGA-3?

Food	Grams Omega-3	Serving Size	Food	Grams Omega-3	Serving Size
Walnuts	1.9	1 ounce	Flounder	0.4	3.5 ounces
Salmon	1.4	3.5 ounces	Crab	0.4	3.5 ounces
Sardines	1.4	3.5 ounces	Shrimp	0.3	3.5 ounces
Canola oil	1.3	1 tablespoon	Cod	0.2	3.5 ounces
Herring	1.2	3.5 ounces	Haddock	0.2	3.5 ounces
Mackerel	1.0	3.5 ounces	Lobster	0.2	3.5 ounces
Trout	0.9	3.5 ounces	Clams	0.2	3.5 ounces
Tuna, fresh	0.8	3.5 ounces	Catfish	0.2	3.5 ounces
Swordfish	0.7	3.5 ounces	Scallops	0.2	3.5 ounces
Tuna, canned	0.5	3.5 ounces			

If you are a fish hater, you can get your omega-3 by taking fish-oil capsules—think cod-liver oil without the taste or smell! These are now available at most pharmacies. Getting enough omega-3 is one of the two big reasons why we all need to eat more fish; the other is because it is the healthiest source of protein available to us. A serving of fish is practically pure protein, with (in some species) a little good fat mixed in for flavor. You get top-quality protein (containing all the amino acids essential for health) without getting the dangerous saturated fat that's always part of the package in land animals. That helps to explain why people in cultures that eat a lot of fish, such as the Japanese, have much lower rates of heart disease than we do, as well as greater life expectancy.

STRATEGIES FOR EATING MORE SEAFOOD

- Order seafood whenever you eat out. Try kinds you've never had before.
- If you think you don't like fish, start with a grilled swordfish or tuna steak. The texture is more meaty than with fish fillets, there are no bones or skin to deal with, and the flavor is every bit as good as a T-bone. A little marinating keeps them juicy.
- Choose tuna in your sandwich for lunch instead of ham or roast beef. The health difference is tremendous!
- Buy precooked shrimp cocktail for a virtually fat-free treat.
- Have the people at the seafood counter in your supermarket cook your lobster for you. They almost all will now, and that takes away 90 percent of the hurdle to having your own lobster.
- Try smoked salmon or mackerel for breakfast. Just remember to spread the cream cheese *very thin*, or skip it altogether.
- Try sushi. It's safe, utterly delicious, and perhaps the healthiest food you can put in your body. (The white rice, however, is not.)

HEALTH FLASH

Do you need a daily multivitamin? It depends on how you eat. If you embrace most of the healthy foods in this book, then you get all the vitamins and minerals you need. Vitamin deficiencies are actually pretty rare in the developed world, and there's little evidence that taking megadoses of particular vitamins helps you at all. In fact, recent studies show that too much vitamin E can be bad for you. The four vitamins hardest to get through diet alone are folic acid, B_6, B_{12}, and D. Folic acid and the B vitamins help keep your heart healthy and may prevent cancer, while vitamin D builds strong bones. Especially if you live in the northern states (and can't get D through sunlight in winter) or are older (and may have trouble absorbing B_{12}), it makes sense to take a multivitamin with 100 percent of the RDA for these four.

WEEK 6   MONDAY

Mission: Let Them Do the Shucking

What do you feel like tonight? Grilled lobster tail? Shrimp on the barbie? Calamari? Choose something healthy yet indulgent and treat yourself right tonight. Plan what you're getting ahead of time so you won't be swayed by naughty temptations. Make it something you know you won't cook at home, because you've got plenty of nights at home to make the healthy food you are comfortable making.

Mission Accomplished? _____

WALK BOX

How Far? _____

Strength Training? _____

How'd It Go? _____

FOOD FOCUS: FRESH SALMON

SUGGESTED RECIPES

Grilled Salmon with Wasabi Cream (p. 215)

Baked Salmon with Apricot Glaze (p. 215)

BREAKFAST_____ LUNCH_____

_____ _____

DINNER_____ SNACKS_____

_____ _____

DRINKS_____ DESSERTS_____

_____ _____

WATER 1 2 3 4 5 6 7 8

NOTES

_____

_____

_____

_____

_____

_____

_____

_____

_____

_____

_____

_____

_____

The Restaurant Habit   Date_____

Mission: Go Splitsville

Don't you always want to sample five different things when you eat out? Here's your chance to do just that. Go out with your main squeeze and get one appetizer and one entrée between you, or pull together three or four of your friends and get a bunch of appetizers and a couple of entrées. Either way, you'll taste a number of different things and have more fun. Make sure you limit your total consumption to less than a full entrée and appetizer. The idea is to eat less, not more!

Mission Accomplished? _____

WALK BOX

HOW FAR? _____

STRENGTH TRAINING? _____

HOW'D IT GO? _____

FOOD FOCUS: LUNCH SALADS

SUGGESTED RECIPES

Key West Crab Salad (p. 204)

Tuscan Tuna and White Bean Salad (p. 198)

BREAKFAST_____ LUNCH_____

_____ _____

DINNER_____ SNACKS_____

_____ _____

DRINKS_____ DESSERTS_____

_____ _____

WATER 1 2 3 4 5 6 7 8

NOTES

_____

_____

_____

_____

_____

_____

_____

_____

_____

_____

_____

_____

_____

The Restaurant Habit   Date_____

WEEK 6   WEDNESDAY

Mission: Shrimpy-Size Me

To develop new habits, you must first do things that feel odd. Fast-food restaurants do an excellent job of designing their menu boards and advertising to make supersizing your meal feel normal and sensible. Today, buck this trend by asking them to shrimpy-size your meal. (No, you don't have to use those exact words.) Order a kid's meal if you feel like it. Do it even if you're convinced it's not enough to fill you up. Eat it, go back to the office or home, look at the clock, and wait one hour to decide if you're still hungry or not. Chances are you won't be, which means you can keep ordering your tiny fast-food meals, knowing you've beaten them at their own game.

Mission Accomplished? _____

WALK BOX

HOW FAR? _____

STRENGTH TRAINING? _____

HOW'D IT GO? _____

FOOD FOCUS: SCALLOPS

SUGGESTED RECIPES

Scallops in Orange Sauce (p. 218)

Caribbean Coconut Scallops (p. 217)

---

172   *Leslie Sansone's Eat Smart, Walk Strong*

BREAKFAST_____ LUNCH_____

_____ _____

DINNER_____ SNACKS_____

_____ _____

DRINKS_____ DESSERTS_____

_____ _____

WATER ① ② ③ ④ ⑤ ⑥ ⑦ ⑧

NOTES

_____

_____

_____

_____

_____

_____

_____

_____

_____

_____

_____

_____

_____

WEEK 6   THURSDAY

Mission: Don't Get Carb-Fooled

I don't recommend calorie counting—I'd rather you develop habits where you eat the right amount of food naturally—but if you're one who treats carbs as if they were rat poison, please check the total number of calories the next time you eat out, whether it's breakfast, lunch, or dinner. Don't let carb-watching be a smoke screen for fat-laden meals! If your typical dinner choice is low on carbs but high in saturated fat from meat or dairy, see what you can order instead that emphasizes fresh veggies and whole grains—and make sure half a stick of butter isn't melted over the fish and veggies before they come!

Mission Accomplished? _____

WALK BOX

HOW FAR? _____

STRENGTH TRAINING? _____

HOW'D IT GO? _____

FOOD FOCUS: SHELLFISH

SUGGESTED RECIPES

Crab-Stuffed Portobello Caps (p. 219)

Tuscan Scallops (p. 219)

BREAKFAST_____ LUNCH_____

_____ _____

DINNER_____ SNACKS_____

_____ _____

DRINKS_____ DESSERTS_____

_____ _____

WATER 1 2 3 4 5 6 7 8

NOTES

_____

_____

_____

_____

_____

_____

_____

_____

_____

_____

_____

_____

The Restaurant Habit

WEEK 6   FRIDAY

Mission: Ban the Buffet

Buffets may as well be designed to break you of any commitment to smart eating. Big vats of unhealthy food lie everywhere, with the unspoken message being "The more you eat, the better value you get!" What a nightmare. Starting today, swear off buffets, brunches, and even all-you-can-eat salad bars (the dressing alone can outcalorie a steak!). It's an easy mission for today, but one with lasting consequences.

Mission Accomplished? _____

WALK BOX

HOW FAR? _____

STRENGTH TRAINING? _____

HOW'D IT GO? _____

FOOD FOCUS: TUNA

SUGGESTED RECIPES

Seared Tuna in Olive Sauce (p. 216)

Nicoise Salad (p. 199)

BREAKFAST_____ LUNCH_____
_____ _____

DINNER_____ SNACKS_____
_____ _____

DRINKS_____ DESSERTS_____
_____ _____

WATER 1 2 3 4 5 6 7 8

NOTES

_____
_____
_____
_____
_____
_____
_____
_____
_____
_____
_____
_____

The Restaurant Habit Date_____

WEEK 6   SATURDAY

Mission: Avoid the Bread Bomb

If you're a low-carb eater, you already know the damage a lot of bread can do to your waistline. If you're not, I'm sorry to break the news to you: Scarfing all the bread in the bread basket before your meal comes will do you no good. Complete with butter or even healthy olive oil, it can add hundreds of calories to your meal. Starting today, when you go out to eat, concentrate on the stuff you really want. Don't even let that bread basket touch your table. After all, you can eat good bread at home anytime you want.

Mission Accomplished? _____

WALK BOX

HOW FAR? _____

STRENGTH TRAINING? _____

HOW'D IT GO? _____

FOOD FOCUS: FISH FOR BREAKFAST

SUGGESTED RECIPES

Scrambled Eggs with Smoked Salmon (p. 192)

Shrimp Frittata (p. 192)

---

178   *Leslie Sansone's Eat Smart, Walk Strong*

BREAKFAST_____ LUNCH_____

_____ _____

DINNER_____ SNACKS_____

_____ _____

DRINKS_____ DESSERTS_____

_____ _____

WATER (1) (2) (3) (4) (5) (6) (7) (8)

NOTES

_____

_____

_____

_____

_____

_____

_____

_____

_____

_____

_____

_____

_____

The Restaurant Habit   Date_____

WEEK 6   SUNDAY WRAP-UP

THE PERFECT SUPPORT SYSTEM

PLANNING

Three smart behaviors I can adopt next week to support my eating goals:

1. _____
2. _____
3. _____

EDUCATION

What I've learned so far:

NEW HABITS	FOOD SOLUTIONS
Intentional Eating	Water
Breakfast	Whole Grains and Legumes
Portion Control	Good Fat
Slow Food	Vegetables
Snack	Fruit
Restaurant	Fish

REPETITION

This week's behaviors:

(Put a ✓ next to those you'll keep doing, an X next to those that weren't useful to you, and an ⟶ next to those that you'll try again later.)

1. ___ Let Them Do the Shucking   4. ___ Don't Get Carb-Fooled
2. ___ Go Splitsville   5. ___ Ban the Buffet
3. ___ Shrimpy-Size Me   6. ___ Avoid the Bread Bomb

Other Restaurant Habits you thought of this week:

_____

_____

Ten behaviors from the past six weeks that are becoming habits:

1. _____ 6. _____
2. _____ 7. _____
3. _____ 8. _____
4. _____ 9. _____
5. _____ 10. _____

FLEXIBILITY

Three ways I can make these habits work better for me:

1. _____
2. _____
3. _____

EXERCISE

Miles/steps walked this week: _____
_____

Other exercise: _____
_____
_____

CELEBRATION!

Three things I'm grateful for this week:

1. _____
2. _____
3. _____

TRANSFORMATION

I surprised myself this week by: _____

NOTES

_____

13. Weeks 7–777 Eating Well for Life

Here we are. After six weeks of trying out new behaviors and learning what works for you, you have developed a beautiful and unique constellation of smart lifestyle habits that fit just right. As these habits become more and more a part of you, they reinforce one another, crowd out any bad habits that try to establish themselves, and make it easier and easier for you to stay healthy and slim.

As you now know, a habit is a behavior that will continue on its own unless something significant comes along to change it. Your challenge is to anticipate things that might throw you off and to make sure your lifestyle doesn't encourage them. It's easy! I probably don't even need to mention many of these things, but we all know what happens to people on most diets, right? They slip. This diet is designed specifically to buck that trend, to get easier the longer you are on it, so you want to make sure you have all your bases covered and are ready for whatever curves life throws at you.

If eating were the only

consideration, I have no doubt that you would continue to succeed, based on what you've done in the past six weeks. But we don't eat in a vacuum, do we? Many other factors impact our life, any of which can spill over and affect our eating habits. In this chapter, I'll list the most common factors that can upset diet, and I'll give you some tips for heading them off at the pass.

1. STRESS

Stress is any perceived threat to your well-being. It can be a snarling dog, the danger of layoffs at your company, or icy winter roads. Whatever the stress factor, it causes physiological reactions in your body in order to help you escape danger. Heart rate and alertness increase as energy gets diverted from functions like digestion and memory (in fact, stress has been shown to suppress short-term memory) to survival tools like muscles and senses. For a brief stretch, you run a little faster and see a little more sharply. But you aren't designed to be on this level of high alert too often. Brief stress now and then causes no health problems; chronic stress causes plenty. It raises blood pressure, wears out heart valves, and makes blockages in our arteries more likely. It also causes many people to overeat, or to become chronic snackers as a way of displacing the stress.

The best way to stay a smart eater is to keep stress at a minimum in your daily life. Here are my favorite tips for doing that:

- **Exercise.** By raising heart rate and flooding your bloodstream with adrenaline, stress primes your body for exercise. You may as well give it what it wants. Exercise is the finest way to burn off stress in a positive manner, one that actually improves health and looks.
- **Sleep.** While you sleep, your body works to remove stress hormones from your blood. If you aren't getting from seven to nine hours of shut-eye, you may never get all that anxiety out of your system.
- **Spirituality.** It's a proven fact that those who trust in a higher power live longer, healthier, and more relaxed lives than those who think they are solely responsible for holding the world together. Find a house of worship or a retreat center that fits your beliefs and see what a difference it can make in your week.
- **Relaxation.** Whether it's yoga, meditation, massage, baths, soothing music, or a stump in the woods, finding a sanctuary for quiet is an important need in all our lives.
- **Don't overcommit.** We all like to say yes. Yes to projects at work, yes to our kids being involved in soccer, track, the yearbook, and student government, yes to dinner with friends. But having too many fun things in one day can make none of them fun. Pace yourself so you keep your stress down and truly enjoy the things you do take on.

- **Reduce your environmental noise.** If your daily surroundings are saturated with TVs, car radios, cell-phone calls, and other distractions, your inner turmoil will quietly grow without you even realizing it. Your life doesn't need a sound track; fewer distractions will allow you to concentrate on one activity at a time, which is the key to doing things well.

2. KIDS

There are certain stages in a woman's life when she is more likely to gain weight, and having children is the biggie. Physiological changes are partially responsible, but this weight gain is primarily due to the changes in lifestyle and eating patterns that occur after childbirth. It's easy to become less active when staying home with a new baby, and sometimes you never get back to your former active self. Don't let that happen. Also, with less free time on your hands, you are more likely to wolf down whatever you can whenever you can. This is understandable when you have an infant, but make sure you get back to normal within a few months. As your kids get older, it becomes more important than ever to establish smart eating habits, because the habits you develop will help them adopt healthy eating patterns for life.

3. DEPRESSION

As I said earlier, overeating bouts are rarely about hunger. Often they are a way of "self-medicating" our mood with comfort foods or a quick sugar rush. Watch out for the dangerous cycle that can develop, where depression leads to overeating and then to weight gain, which adds to depression. At the first sign of this cycle, act quickly to break the pattern. Many mild forms of depression can be relieved by exercise. Lack of sleep is another classic cause. You may feel like you operate fine on six hours of sleep, until you realize you've been down for months. Stress, of course, is another factor. Try making some lifestyle adjustments to improve your mood; if that doesn't work, talk with your doctor about how to turn life around before the depression and overeating become more serious.

4. FRIENDS—FRIENDLY AND OTHERWISE

Friends and family can be the strongest supports to weight-loss goals. They can also trip you up. Do those in your social network encourage you to walk, or to treat yourself to a piece of cake "just this once" because you deserve it? Assembling a team of buddies who will help you walk the walk is critical to your success; very few people manage to eat smart when others in their lives constantly belittle their goals or make food for them that they shouldn't eat. Make sure your special people know how important your goals are to you, and ask them to help you in whatever small ways they can. They'll be happy to do so; then they can share in your triumphs along the way.

5. THE CREEPING SNACK MONSTER

Snacking is playing with fire. It can be a useful tool, but it's easy to get burned. That's why I'm generally against snacking; I've seen too many people start off snacking wisely, then creep toward larger and more frequent snacks, until they are eating the equivalent of two extra meals a day. If you've been snacking, this might be a good time to phase it out slowly. If you find that snacking is really helping you meet your weight goals, then by all means keep doing it, but make sure to keep those snacks to a couple of hundred calories each.

6. MONTHLY MENSTRUAL CYCLES

I'm sure you already know how your natural rhythms affect your hunger and cravings. The important thing is to recognize these cravings for what they are and to keep in mind that this is perfectly natural. Don't fight your body. It's okay to indulge cravings on occasion if that helps you to stay on track the rest of the time. Just make sure that listening to "body wisdom" doesn't become an excuse to cut loose with the chips and dip!

7. CHANGING SEASONS

The reaction to seasonal change is as old as life itself. Summer turns to autumn, leaves disappear in a blast of cold north wind, we move inside, and our thoughts turn to meat dripping over an open fire and steaming mugs of hot chocolate. Something in our brains wants to hibernate—and to put on ten pounds of fat before we do! It's only natural for us to gain a few pounds in winter, when we are less active, and then lose them again in summer. The danger is that we may gain the winter pounds and forget to lose the summer pounds. That's why it's best not to gain the winter pounds at all. Indoor walking is the best way I know to fight off Old Man Winter and keep yourself active throughout the year. If you find yourself sleepier and more sluggish in winter, try using some full-spectrum lightbulbs in your house, which give you summerlike light in the dark of December.

8. AGE

In America, we believe it's almost automatic that we'll put on a few pounds in middle age and a few more as we get older. Not only is this not automatic; it's dangerous. All the diseases we've discussed in this book increase in direct proportion to late-life weight gain. And it isn't automatic. In most of the world, people expect to maintain their weight throughout adulthood. Most Americans, however, tend to become less active as they get older, and that's where the weight gain comes from.

True, our metabolisms slow down a bit as we age, but that can be reversed through exercise. Keep walking into your eighties and you'll maintain the metabolism of a thirty-year-old. You'll have the health of one, too!

BLESSINGS ON YOU

You now have everything you need for a lifetime of healthy and joyful experience with food. In fact, you had everything you needed all along. Our bodies have a natural attraction to healthy food, as well as to being physically active. It's just a matter of getting in touch with our core and fending off the daily bombardment of misinformation that seeks to make us act against our instincts. I hope this plan has helped you get reacquainted with those instincts. Letting them guide you, you need never feel guilty about eating again. Next time you say a blessing before a meal, feel that blessing reflected right back upon you. Eating is a sacred act. Every time you do it, you reconnect with the source of all that is sacred.

PART III

RECIPES FOR LIFE

14. Breakfast

Blueberry Breakfast Smoothie

For those turned off by solid food in the morning, a smoothie is the perfect answer. Sweet and delicious, it's made high-protein by the use of yogurt, skim milk, or silken tofu. If you haven't tried silken tofu, which adds a smooth creaminess to any drink, start there. In addition to 5 grams of protein per serving, this smoothie is absolutely packed with fiber, vitamin C, potassium, and antioxidants. Bottoms up!

2 cups fresh or frozen blueberries
8 ounces silken tofu
1 large banana, peeled
1 cup apple juice

Combine all ingredients in a blender and blend until smooth. Drink up.

Serves 2 as breakfast

Orange Mango Smoothie

Picture yourself on a veranda in Barbados as you sip this tropical smoothie. Even in the dead of a northern winter, it will get your day off to a bright start. Feel free to substitute other fruits for the mango, or soy milk for the yogurt.

2 cups fresh or frozen mango
1 cup vanilla yogurt
1 large banana, peeled
1 cup orange juice

Combine all ingredients in a blender and blend until smooth. Serve immediately or store in the refrigerator.

Serves 2 as breakfast

Cranberry-Almond Granola

Making your own granola is easier than you can imagine! And when you make it yourself, you can be sure it isn't too sweet and that it has lots of goodies, like the almonds and dried cranberries in this batch. Feel free to substitute other nuts for the almonds, or raisins for the cranberries.

3 cups old-fashioned oats
1 cup slivered almonds
1/2 cup coconut (optional)
1/3 cup honey

1/4 cup canola oil
1 cup dried cranberries
1/2 cup dried banana chips (optional)

1. Preheat the oven to 325°F.
2. Stir together the oats, almonds, coconut, honey, and oil in a large bowl.
3. Spread the mixture in a high-sided baking pan and bake until the oats are golden (about 30 minutes). Remember to stir the mixture every few minutes to prevent sticking.
4. Remove from the oven, let cool, and then stir in the cranberries and banana chips. Store in an airtight container.

Makes 6 1/2 cups; serves about 12

Cinnamon-Walnut Muffins

Here's a dangerous recipe to put in your hands. Muffins are high in calories, so you don't get to eat half a batch for breakfast. These are packed with nutrients and have more protein than most muffins because of the walnuts. The cinnamon is an important ingredient because cinnamon has a magical ability to reduce insulin resistance and regulate blood sugar. One muffin with a nice piece of fruit makes a healthful breakfast.

1 cup white flour
1 cup whole-wheat flour
2 teaspoons baking powder
2 teaspoons cinnamon
1/4 teaspoon salt
1/2 cup sugar

2 eggs
1/4 cup canola oil
1 cup milk
1 cup grated apple, carrot, or zucchini, peeled
1/2 cup walnuts, chopped

1. Preheat the oven to 400°F.
2. Grease a 12-cup muffin tin.
3. Place the dry ingredients—both kinds of flour, baking powder, cinnamon, salt, and sugar—in a large bowl and mix together.
4. Place the wet ingredients—eggs, canola oil, milk, and grated fruit or veggie—in a separate bowl and mix together.
5. Pour the wet ingredients into the dry and mix briefly. Don't overmix, as that makes the batter tough. It's okay if there are still some lumps.

6. Fold the walnuts in.

7. Divide the batter evenly among the muffin cups and bake in the oven for 18 to 20 minutes or until golden brown.

8. Remove from the oven and let sit for several minutes before taking the muffins out of the tin.

Makes 12 muffins

Nutty Pancakes

These pancakes may be nutty, but they sure aren't crazy! With extra protein and flavor from the almonds, they make a very sane breakfast. Use less syrup than you think you need; a drizzle of sweetness is usually enough, and it lets the almondy flavor come through.

1 cup whole-wheat flour
1 cup unbleached flour
2 teaspoons baking powder
1/2 cup ground almonds
1/2 teaspoon salt
1 teaspoon cinnamon
2 eggs
2 cups milk
1 tablespoon canola oil, plus more for cooking
1 teaspoon almond extract

1. Place the dry ingredients—both kinds of flour, baking powder, ground almonds, salt, and cinnamon—in a large bowl and mix together.

2. Place the wet ingredients—eggs, milk, canola oil, and almond extract—in a separate bowl and mix together.

3. Pour the wet ingredients over the dry ingredients and mix until just blended. It's better to have some lumps (which will cook out) than to overmix the batter and end up with tough pancakes.

4. Heat a large nonstick skillet over medium heat, pour half a teaspoon of canola oil into it (if your nonstick skillet is in good shape, you might not need this), and pour one ladleful of batter into the skillet. Cook until bubbles form over the top of the pancake and the edges look dry (about 2 minutes).

5. Flip the pancake with a spatula, cook the underside about 30 seconds, and serve at once with warm maple syrup.

Makes 12 6-inch pancakes

Scrambled Eggs with Smoked Salmon

A great way to please a crowd at breakfast!

  6 eggs, beaten
  3 ounces smoked salmon, cut in small pieces
  1 tablespoon fresh dill, minced (optional)
  2 ounces low-fat cream cheese
  2 tablespoons butter

1. Combine the eggs, salmon, and dill in a large bowl. Using a knife, flick bits of the cream cheese into the eggs and mix well.
2. Heat the butter in a large skillet over medium heat, until sizzling. Add the egg mixture and cook, stirring slowly, until the eggs are set but not dry (about 3 minutes). Serve immediately.

Serves 4

Shrimp Frittata

Breakfast, lunch, or dinner, you can't go wrong with this tasty dish. Frittatas are omelettes that are finished off open-faced under the broiler instead of being folded in half. The result is puffier and drier than a regular omelette. The frittata can be cut into squares or wedges, which makes this an ideal brunch food, too!

  4 eggs, beaten
  8 ounces cooked and peeled shrimp
  2 green onions, chopped
  1 tablespoon soy sauce
  1/2 red pepper, stemmed, seeded, and diced (optional)
  1/2 teaspoon pepper
  1 tablespoon canola oil
  1 tablespoon Parmesan cheese

1. Preheat the broiler.
2. Place the eggs, shrimp, green onions, soy sauce, red pepper, and pepper in a large bowl and mix together.
3. Heat the canola oil in an ovenproof skillet over medium heat. Add the egg mixture and cook until the bottom is set but the top is still runny (about 2 minutes).
4. Sprinkle Parmesan cheese on top and place the skillet under the broiler. Broil until the top of the frittata is golden and bubbly (about 2 minutes). Serve at once.

Serves 2 to 4

Fried Eggs on Garlic Toast

The Italians have created a whole cuisine that basically revolves around stale bread. They use stale bread as an ingredient in soups, pasta, salads, and bruschetta, of course. Here is another idea that will open up new possibilities. Instead of dipping your toast in fried eggs, fry your eggs over the toast. You get better flavor, better crunch, and you can easily mix in a variety of vegetables, from garlic (as in this version) to mushrooms, asparagus, onion, or peppers. The salsa is optional.

4 slices multigrain bread, diced
1 teaspoon minced garlic
1/4 cup olive oil, plus 1 tablespoon
4 eggs
1/2 cup salsa

1. Place the diced bread and the garlic in a large bowl and mix together. Add 1/4 cup oil and stir the ingredients together.
2. Place a large nonstick skillet over medium heat and then add the bread and garlic mixture. Cook, stirring, until it begins to sizzle and brown.
3. Add the tablespoon of oil to the pan (around the bread) and heat for 10 seconds. Then crack the eggs on top of the bread and cook until the eggs set (about 2 minutes). If desired, flip and cook for 30 seconds more.
4. Remove the eggs and bread to individual serving plates and add the salsa to the skillet. Cook until hot and bubbling; then pour over the eggs. Serve immediately.

Serves 2 to 4

Spinach and Chèvre Omelette

Omelettes are much easier to make than most people think. The trick is to do less, not more. The ultimate breakfast food, they contain enough protein, fat, vitamins, and fiber to keep you focused and snack-free till lunch. They also make a great light dinner. From start to finish, an omelette takes less than 5 minutes, so have all your fillings ready to go. The combination of spinach or chard and tangy chèvre (goat cheese) is magical, but the possibilities are unlimited. Some particularly delightful combos are listed at the end of this recipe, but use your imagination and invent something brand-new. This makes a fairly large omelette for one; by adding a third egg, you can easily make an omelette large enough for two people to split.

2 eggs
1/4 teaspoon salt
1/4 teaspoon pepper
1 teaspoon canola oil
2 ounces chèvre
1/2 cup cooked spinach or chard, chopped

1. Place the eggs in a bowl, add the salt and pepper, and beat together with a fork.
2. Heat the canola oil over medium heat in a large nonstick skillet until hot but not smoking.
3. Add the eggs and let them spread over the bottom of the pan. You don't need to touch them with any implement. If they don't cover the bottom, you can tilt the pan slightly to help them out.
4. When the eggs have set (perhaps a minute or two), crumble the chèvre over them evenly. Then spread the spinach or chard over the top.
5. Cook for another minute or so, until the cheese has melted and the eggs are completely set. Using a spatula, fold the omelette in half. Serve immediately.

Makes 1 omelette

Use omelettes as a way to get your vegetables in at breakfast and to use up leftovers. Most veggies will need to be sautéed briefly in oil before you make the omelette. Some good omelette fillings:

- Ham, green onions, and Swiss cheese
- Tomatoes, Brie, and basil
- Cooked broccoli and Monterey Jack
- Smoked chicken and Gouda
- Mushrooms and cheddar
- Zucchini, sun-dried tomatoes, and feta
- Smoked salmon, green onions, and cream cheese
- Leftover Spinach with Roasted Garlic Cream (p. 231)
- Leftover Rainbow Pepper Medley (p. 228)

15. SANDWICHES AND WRAPS

Cranberry-Orange Turkey Sandwich

Light, bright fruit flavors go surprisingly well with turkey. We tend to take advantage of this only at Thanksgiving, but here's another chance. The nuttiness of multigrain bread is perfect with this, but you could use a wrap to cut down on carbs if you prefer. The peppery arugula greens are essential to offset the sweetness of the other ingredients. The beautiful colors of this dish would also make a great salad! Skip the bread, mix the arugula with milder greens, use dried cranberries instead of cranberry sauce, and throw in some walnuts and Easy Buttermilk Dressing (p. 206). Yum!

2 slices multigrain bread
1 teaspoon mayonnaise
1 tablespoon cranberry sauce

2 slices turkey breast
1 handful arugula greens
4 to 6 sections orange or clementine

1. Spread the mayonnaise on one slice of bread and the cranberry sauce on the other.
2. Place the turkey, arugula, and citrus sections on top of the cranberry sauce. Close the mayo slice over the top to make a sandwich.

Makes 1 sandwich

Turkey Pesto Wrap

The eye-popping flavor of pesto makes it the best sandwich condiment in the world. You can even skip the cheese when pesto's on the scene. Combine it with sliced turkey breast and a whole-wheat tortilla for a high-protein, low-carb, vitamin-rich lunch that will keep you humming for hours.

1 whole-wheat tortilla
1 tablespoon homemade Pesto (p. 236), or store-bought
2 slices turkey breast

1/2 carrot, shredded or thinly sliced
Other veggies of choice

1. Spread the pesto evenly over the tortilla.
2. Layer the turkey over the pesto.
3. Sprinkle with the carrot or any other vegetables you like.
4. Wrap your sandwich up like you fold a burrito (sides in, bottom up, top down). Devour!

Makes 1 sandwich

Pork Tenderloin Sandwich

Plan on making this sandwich the day after you've made the Cumin and Orange–Scented Pork Loin (p. 225) for dinner. Leftover pork slices deliver a taste no cold-cut can match. By using orange slices to accentuate the orange flavor already in the pork, you get a sandwich bursting with freshness. Getting away from the cheese is the key to turning a sandwich into an extremely healthy lunch. Sprouts are available in all supermarkets, and they contain one of the most intense concentrations of vitamins you can find. (Some variations: Use a whole-wheat wrap or tortilla instead of bread, or skip the orange and use a pickle.)

2 slices multigrain bread, toasted if you like
1 tablespoon mayonnaise
2 slices boneless pork loin

1 slice orange, peeled (about 1/4-inch thick)
1 small handful sprouts

Spread the mayonnaise on a slice of bread. Add the pork and orange on top of the bread. Top with the sprouts and second bread slice; then cut in half and serve.

Makes 1 sandwich

New PB&J Sandwich

That old standby, peanut butter and jelly, actually has some nutritional merit to it, but let's face it, it's not very interesting. This sandwich solves that problem. We know that peanut butter and jelly go well together, right? And we've all seen those chicken or beef skewers with spicy peanut sauce around, right? This sandwich combines those ideas and adds some cuke for crunch. All these ingredients (except the bread) are common ingredients in Asian cooking, so this really isn't as strange a combination as it seems. Feel free to substitute another jelly for the hot pepper if you don't want the spice, and you can skip the soy sauce if you prefer. Once you've tried this, the wheels will start turning in your head, and you'll think up lots of other ways to reinvent the sandwich and keep lunch fun.

2 tablespoons natural peanut butter
1 teaspoon soy sauce
2 slices multigrain bread, toasted if you like
4 slices cucumber

2 slices turkey breast
1 tablespoon cilantro, chopped (optional)
1 tablespoon hot-pepper jelly

1. Scoop the peanut butter into a bowl and mix the soy sauce into it. Spread this on one slice of bread. Press the cucumber slices onto this and cover with the turkey slices. Sprinkle with cilantro, if desired.
2. Spread the hot-pepper jelly on the other slice of bread and close this over the turkey side. Cut in half and eat.

Makes 1 sandwich

16. SALADS AND DRESSINGS

Black Bean, Orange, and Cucumber Salad

Black beans and oranges make a surprisingly wonderful combination and can serve a variety of uses. This no-cook side salad has a Latin American feel and goes well with any cuisine from that part of the world, especially if it features fish or pork.

    1/4 cup extra-virgin olive oil
    Juice of 1/2 lime
    1 clove garlic, pressed
    1 teaspoon salt
    2 15-ounce cans black beans, drained
    1 large cucumber, peeled and diced
    2 large oranges, peeled and diced

1. Combine the olive oil, lime juice, garlic, and salt in a large bowl. Mix.
2. Add the beans, cucumber, and oranges, toss gently so as not to break up the beans, and serve.

Serves 6 to 8

Surprise Beet-Mango Salad

This recipe actually has a few surprises in it. For one, the beets are—surprise!—canned. Raw beets are a pain to work with. They need to be boiled for a long time, and then you have to try to slip their burning-hot skins off. Whichever way you cut it, you risk staining every surface you use beet red (or purple). And you know what? The canned ones taste just as good. Shhh, don't tell any gourmet cooks out there; they might get mad. Just quietly make this salad and enjoy.

    1 15-ounce can sliced beets, drained
    1 fresh mango, peeled, pitted, and cubed, or 10 ounces jarred mango
    1/2 cup extra-virgin olive oil
    Juice of 1/4 lemon
    1/2 teaspoon salt

Place the beets, mango, olive oil, lemon juice, and salt in a large bowl. Toss and serve. (Don't worry if the mango turns pink.)

Serves 4

Spanish Tuna and Chickpea Salad

Chickpeas are a cooking staple in all the Mediterranean cultures, from Spain and Italy to North Africa and the Middle East. Like other legumes, they are superhigh in fiber and superlow in calories. This salad's main ingredients–chickpeas, oranges, artichoke hearts, and fish–capture some of the essence of Spanish cooking. This dish would be equally scrumptious with shredded chicken, shrimp, or sardines.

8 ounces washed greens (romaine lettuce works well)
1 15-ounce can chickpeas, drained
1 6-ounce can tuna, drained
1 orange, peeled, seeded, and chopped
2 thin slices red onion
1 6-ounce jar marinated artichoke hearts, drained
1/2 cup No-Fail Vinaigrette (p. 205)

1. Arrange the greens on the bottom of four salad bowls (or use plates).
2. Combine the chickpeas, tuna, orange, onion, and artichoke hearts in a large bowl. Pour the vinaigrette over the top and toss gently to combine.
3. Spoon some of the mixture onto the greens in each bowl and serve.

Serves 4

Tuscan Tuna and White Bean Salad

If you think healthier cooking means hours of prep, this dish will teach you otherwise. It's ready in minutes, incredibly healthy, and can fill several roles. Use it as a first course, a lunch side dish, or serve it on a bed of greens, along with crusty bread and a glass of red wine, for a delightful light dinner. By changing the ingredients somewhat, you can make weekly variations on this and keep it interesting. Some of the ingredients you might add: fresh tomato, rosemary, basil, anchovies, roasted red peppers, or black olives.

1 15-ounce can white beans, drained
1 6-ounce can tuna, drained
4 sun-dried tomatoes preserved in oil, drained and minced
2 tablespoons red onion, minced (optional)

1/4 cup extra-virgin olive oil
1 tablespoon lemon juice
Salt and pepper

1. Combine the beans, tuna, sun-dried tomatoes, and onion in a large serving bowl.
2. Pour the olive oil over the salad and toss to coat, being gentle so that the beans do not break up.
3. Add the lemon juice, salt and pepper to taste, and toss gently again. Serve immediately.

Serves 4 as a first course or 2 as an entrée

Tuna and Radish Salad with Creamy Avocado Dressing

People don't eat enough radishes, mostly because we don't see many recipes that include them. But radishes are very healthy and very versatile. They work best when their heat can be softened by something creamy, as in this salad. Romaine works well as the green here. Try this with crabmeat or chicken breast, too.

    4 cups washed greens
    1 6-ounce can tuna, drained
    1/2 cup Creamy Avocado Dressing (p. 205)
    4 radishes, sliced thin

1. Arrange the greens on the bottom of four salad bowls (or use plates).
2. Flake the tuna and divide it evenly over the greens.
3. Pour the dressing over the salads.
4. Sprinkle the radish slices over the top.

Serves 4 as a side salad or 2 as an entrée

Nicoise Salad

Nicoise salad is a gem because it's so easy and because it contains a delectable combination of vegetables, healthy fats, and protein. You could live on Nicoise salad alone, and it would be a pretty good life. This recipe skips the traditional boiled potatoes in order to make it a low-carb dish, but feel free to add a FEW.

    1 pound green beans, ends trimmed
    10 ounces washed greens (romaine works well)
    2 large tomatoes, cut in wedges
    1 6-ounce can tuna, drained
    2 hard-boiled eggs, quartered
    1/2 cup No-Fail Vinaigrette (p. 205)
    1/2 cup Greek olives
    1 tablespoon capers (optional)

1. Steam the green beans in a covered pot until tender but still crisp (about 8 minutes). Dunk them in a pot of cold water to cool them.
2. Arrange the greens on a large bowl or platter.
3. Pile the tomatoes, tuna, eggs, and green beans on top of the lettuce.
4. Drizzle the dressing over the salad.
5. Sprinkle the olives and capers over the top. Serve at once.

Serves 4 as a first course or 2 as an entrée

Wilted Spinach Salad with Bacon

By no stretch of the imagination is bacon healthy. Does that mean you have to give it up entirely? No! Using little bits of "bad stuff" here and there will give you much more flexibility in your diet and will prevent you from feeling deprived, while doing minimal damage to your waistline. This salad is a good example, with a tiny bit of bacon divided four ways giving you that wonderful smoky flavor. Wilted salads used to be popular, and there are some signs that they may become so again. They work particularly well with spinach, because wilting the leaves takes that raw spinach edge away while preserving the fresh crunch. Wilted salads seem to call out for a little sweetness, provided here by the balsamic vinegar and maple syrup.

2 slices bacon
6 ounces washed spinach
2 tablespoons olive oil
1 tablespoon balsamic vinegar
1 teaspoon maple syrup or honey
1 hard-boiled egg, chopped
1 tablespoon minced red onion
Salt and pepper

1. Place the bacon slices between paper towels, put on a plate, and cook on high in the microwave for 2 minutes, or until crisp. Set aside to drain.
2. Place the spinach leaves and hard-boiled egg in a large serving bowl.
3. Warm the oil in a skillet over medium heat. Add the vinegar, maple syrup, and onion and stir to combine. Immediately pour this over the spinach and toss gently.
4. Season with salt and pepper, crumble bacon over the top, and serve at once.

Serves 2 to 4 as a side salad

Garden of Eden Pasta Salad

Raw vegetables are unparalleled in their health benefits. They retain all their vitamins and enzymes (some of which are generally lost when vegetables are cooked) and provide lots of roughage to keep your insulin response low. They also make any dish easier, since there's less cooking! The key to making this pasta salad appealing is to chop or finely dice the raw veggies, so that no one is stuck gnawing on half a tree of broccoli. Feel free to throw in leftover chicken or ham to up the protein content. Penne or farfalle (bow ties) are good pasta shapes for this dish.

1/2 cup extra-virgin olive oil
1/4 cup fresh basil, minced
2 tablespoons balsamic vinegar
1 tablespoon minced garlic
1/2 teaspoon salt
8 ounces short pasta of your choice, cooked
1 head broccoli florets, chopped in small pieces
1 package cherry tomatoes, halved
2 ounces black olives, pitted and chopped
4 ounces feta cheese, diced
1 yellow pepper, seeded and diced
1 avocado, peeled, pitted, and diced

1. Combine the olive oil, basil, balsamic vinegar, garlic, and salt in a bowl or container and whisk or shake until well blended.
2. Combine all other ingredients in a large bowl. Pour the dressing over the top and toss. Serve immediately, or refrigerate for up to 2 days.

Serves 6 to 8

Prosciutto, Fig, and Melon Salad

Flavors pop in all directions in this salad. Salty, sweet, savory, bitter—you name it. The key is the prosciutto, a cured ham from Italy that's very salty, so you eat it in paper-thin slices as a flavoring with other foods. Almost all delis carry prosciutto these days.

2 thin slices prosciutto, cut into 1/4-inch strips
8 dried figs, quartered, stems removed
8 ounces cantaloupe or other melon, cubed
6 ounces arugula or other washed greens
1/4 cup walnuts, chopped
1/4 cup extra-virgin olive oil
1 tablespoon balsamic vinegar

1. Combine the prosciutto, figs, melon, arugula, and walnuts in a large bowl. Toss with the olive oil and balsamic vinegar. Serve.

Serves 4 as a first course

Chicken, Pear, Pecan, and Blue Cheese Salad

This classic salad becomes a main course with the addition of chicken. Any leftover chicken works, though grilled chicken is especially good. You can even use diced turkey breast from the deli. A nice bitter green offsets the sweetness of the pear and pecans. In springtime, you can use tender young dandelion greens straight from your yard (provided it's free of fertilizer and pesticides); otherwise, try arugula.

5 ounces washed greens
2 ounces arugula or dandelion greens, washed and chopped
2 cups cooked chicken meat
1/2 cup pecans
4 ounces blue cheese, crumbled
1 ripe Anjou pear, cored and sliced
1/2 cup No-Fail Vinaigrette (p. 205)

1. Preheat the oven to 350°F. (a toaster oven works well) and toast the pecans until golden and sizzling (about 5 minutes). Remove from oven.
2. Combine all ingredients in a large serving bowl and then toss to mix. Serve at once.

Serves 6 as a first course

Blackened Chicken Salad

Guys gravitate to grills like moths to a flame, but for some reason many women aren't comfortable using them. That's changing as we discover how incredibly easy and fun grilling really is. Grills are fast and allow fat to cook off, keeping calories low. If you can use an oven, you can use a grill. Try it this week!

The chicken:

2 pounds boneless, skinless chicken breasts
1/2 cup Easy Buttermilk Dressing (p. 206), or store-bought dressing
2 tablespoons blackened or Cajun seasoning

The salad:

10 ounces washed greens
1 large ripe tomato, cut in wedges
1/2 cup Easy Buttermilk Dressing (p. 206), or store-bought dressing

1. Marinate the chicken in 1/2 cup of the dressing for at least 2 hours in the refrigerator.
2. Turn the grill to high heat.
3. Remove the chicken from the marinade, sprinkle it with the blackened seasoning, and grill about 5 minutes on each side, until chicken is white all the way through. Remove from heat.
4. Arrange the greens on individual salad plates and top with the tomato.
5. Slice the chicken in strips and place it on top of the salads. Pour dressing over the top and serve.

Serves 6

South of France Chicken Salad

Why make chicken salad with mayo when olive oil makes it more delicious and very healthy? For best flavor, buy boneless chicken breasts and sauté them in olive oil for 4 minutes per side. But for ease, just get a thick slab of cooked chicken or turkey breast from the deli counter. If you've never used capers, you'll be amazed at the way they perk up any dish!

1 pound cooked chicken or turkey breast, roughly chopped
2 celery stalks, diced
12 cherry tomatoes, halved
12 Greek olives (pitted if you prefer)
1 tablespoon capers, drained
6 sprigs fresh thyme or oregano, minced

1/2 cup extra-virgin olive oil
Juice of 1/4 lemon
Salt and pepper to taste

1. Combine the chicken, celery, tomatoes, olives, capers, and thyme or oregano in a large bowl.
2. Pour in the olive oil and mix.
3. Squeeze the lemon juice over the top and mix again.
4. Season to taste with salt and pepper and serve.

Serves 4

Key West Crab Salad

In Florida, they do wonderful things with crab, using some of their bountiful local produce to create a variety of delicacies. Here, creamy avocado and sweet-sour orange team up with crab for a tropical salad that will make you dream of sunsets in Key West. For a true Key West experience, serve with fresh Cuban bread and a tall mango iced tea. (If crabmeat is too expensive where you live, feel free to substitute cooked shrimp or canned tuna.)

1/3 cup extra-virgin olive oil
2 tablespoons orange juice
1 tablespoon lime juice
1 teaspoon minced garlic
1/2 teaspoon salt
10 ounces mixed greens

6 ounces crabmeat
1 large avocado, peeled, pitted, and diced
1 6-ounce jar marinated artichoke hearts, drained and chopped
1 large ripe tomato, cut in wedges
2 tablespoons cilantro, minced (optional)

1. To make the vinaigrette, combine the olive oil, orange juice, lime juice, garlic, and salt in a bowl or small container and whisk or shake until well blended.
2. Combine the other ingredients in a large serving bowl, toss gently with the vinaigrette, and serve.

Serves 4

No-Fail Vinaigrette

Making a spectacular vinaigrette is so easy, it's a wonder that people buy bottled dressing. The thing almost everyone does wrong when they make dressing is not adding enough salt. It's the salt that makes the salad greens come to life. (Don't overdo it, and watch your salt intake if you have high blood pressure or a salt-sensitive condition.) This vinaigrette lasts forever in your cupboard, so make a big batch and use it regularly. Some variations: Use balsamic vinegar instead of lemon juice if you want a deeper, sweeter flavor. Add any fresh herb you like. And add 1 tablespoon of mustard for extra bite. Or, for a creamy vinaigrette, put all the ingredients below into a food processor, add 3 tablespoons of mayonnaise, and blend until smooth.

1 cup extra-virgin olive oil
Juice of 1 lemon
1 teaspoon salt
1 teaspoon pepper
1 teaspoon minced garlic (optional)

Place all the ingredients into a glass or Tupperware container with a lid, cover, and shake until blended. Store in the cupboard (refrigerate if you've added mustard or mayonnaise). Remember to shake before using.

Makes 1 cup

Creamy Avocado Dressing

Here's a luxurious way to dress salads in good, heart-healthy fat. It also makes a great sauce for veggies, meat, fish, or Mexican dishes. Best of all, it's ready in seconds!

1 large avocado, peeled and pitted
1/4 cup extra-virgin olive oil
Juice of 1/2 lemon
1/2 teaspoon salt
1 teaspoon minced garlic
1/2 cup water

1. Combine all ingredients except the water in a blender or food processor. Blend until smooth.
2. With the machine running, slowly add the water until a creamy dressinglike consistency has been reached. You may not need all the water. Serve immediately or chill before serving.

Makes enough to dress a large salad for 8

Easy Buttermilk Dressing

Buttermilk is a great secret ingredient, because it makes things creamy and savory without adding fat. If you have a blender or food processor, you'll discover just how easy buttermilk or ranch dressing is to make, and you'll never buy store-bought again! Add capers, anchovies, or mustard for a saltier dressing, or 1/4 cup honey for a sweeter one.

3/4 cup buttermilk
1/2 cup chopped onion
1 clove garlic (or 1 teaspoon minced)
3/4 cup mayonnaise
1/2 teaspoon salt
1/2 teaspoon pepper
1 teaspoon fresh dill (optional)

Combine all ingredients in a blender or food processor. Blend until smooth and creamy. Store in an airtight jar in the refrigerator.

Makes 2 cups

17. SOUPS AND STEWS

Apricot Lentil Stew

The key to this recipe is the dried apricots. They plump up nicely in the soup and add a wonderful sweetness to the hearty lentils. Combined with the spices, they give this dish an eye-opening flavor you don't expect from lentil stew. All in all, this is a wonderful source of protein, fiber, and vitamins. Unlike other dried legumes, lentils cook relatively quickly and don't need to be presoaked.

3 tablespoons olive or canola oil
2 onions, peeled and diced
2 carrots, peeled and diced
2 celery stalks, chopped
1 tablespoon cumin
3 cups chicken or vegetable broth
3 cups water
2 cups dried lentils
1 medium eggplant, diced
1 cup dried apricots, chopped
1 teaspoon cinnamon
1 14-ounce can diced tomatoes with juice
1/4 cup fresh parsley, chopped
1/4 cup fresh mint, chopped (optional)
Salt

1. Pour the oil into a large pot over medium heat. Add the onions, carrots, and celery, and sauté until the onions are soft (about 2 minutes).
2. Add the cumin and stir for 15 seconds.
3. Add the broth, water, lentils, eggplant, apricots, cinnamon, and tomatoes. Bring the mixture to a boil; then lower the heat and simmer, covered, until the lentils are tender (about 40 minutes).
4. Add the parsley and mint, stir, and then simmer for an additional 5 minutes. Add salt to taste before serving.

Serves 8

Black Bean and Avocado Chili

This gloriously easy dish is just the one to make when you need dinner in 20 minutes and there's nothing but cans in the house. That sainted combination of black beans, lime, and salt really comes through. You can make it without the avocado, but the avocado makes it creamy and rich without the need for cheese or sour cream, both of which are loaded with saturated fat. Make sure the avocado is nice and ripe. If the idea of all-veggie chili doesn't appeal to you, feel free to mix in a pound of ground turkey or very lean ground beef (you can sauté the meat after the onions and garlic).

2 teaspoons olive or canola oil
1 onion, peeled and diced
1 teaspoon minced garlic
1 14-ounce can diced tomatoes with their juice
2 15-ounce cans black beans, drained
1/2 cup frozen corn kernels
1 tablespoon chili powder
1 teaspoon salt
Juice of 1/2 lime
1 avocado, peeled, pitted, and diced

Garnishes:
Cilantro, minced
Monterey Jack, grated
Hot sauce

1. Heat the oil over medium heat in a large pot.
2. Add the onion and garlic and sauté until soft.
3. Add the tomatoes and juice, beans, corn, chili powder, and salt. Squeeze the lime juice into the pot. Simmer for 10 minutes.
4. Add the avocado and simmer for 5 more minutes.
5. Serve and let people garnish their individual bowls with cilantro, cheese, and hot sauce.

Serves 6

Smoky Fish Chowder

The fish chowder and clam chowder you find in restaurants is anything but healthy. That gluey white paste you could spackle your wall with is filled with flour, butter, and cheap oil. Real New England chowder, however, is plenty good for you. Brimming with onions and fish, and cooked in milk, it'll keep you warm through any cold winter night, just as it has done for generations of fishermen. A little smoked salmon gives this dish a wonderful hint of smokiness that will make you throw out any other chowder recipe you have.

1 tablespoon canola oil
1 onion, peeled and diced
2 large potatoes, peeled and diced
2 stalks celery, diced
1/2 cup fish or vegetable broth
2 pounds cod or other whitefish fillets, cut in chunks
2 cups milk of your choice
4 ounces smoked salmon, flaked
Salt and pepper to taste

1. Heat the canola oil in a large soup pot. Add the onion and cook until soft.
2. Add the potatoes and celery to the pan. Then add the broth, bring to a boil, cover, and simmer the vegetables over low heat until they are soft (about 10 minutes).
3. Add the fish to the vegetables, cover, and simmer until the fish becomes opaque (about 5 minutes).
4. Add the milk and simmer over as low a flame as possible for 30 minutes.
5. Turn off the heat and stir in the smoked salmon. Season with salt and pepper to taste. For best flavor, let the soup sit for at least an hour before serving (though it will be at its best the next day).

Serves 6 as a main dish

18. PASTA

Linguine with Pesto

This is the classic way to serve pesto in Italy. You can substitute any pasta shape you like, except spaghetti or angel hair, which tend to get too gloopy with thick sauces. You can also add grilled zucchini and chicken breast to increase the veggie and protein content. Try egg pasta or whole-wheat pasta for a slower insulin response.

　1 pound dried linguine
　2 cups pesto (p. 236)

1. Bring a large pot of water to a boil.
2. Add the pasta and cook at a rolling boil until just tender. Drain.
3. Mix the pesto with the pasta and serve at once.

Serves 6

Fusilli with Smoked Turkey and Roasted Veggies

Fusilli (corkscrews) is one of the most fun pasta shapes. It also holds sauce well. In winter, make this sauce with the roasted tomatoes and onions, as described, for some warming comfort food. In summer, substitute sun-dried tomatoes for the roasted vegetables so you don't have to use the oven, and serve at room temperature.

　1 Roasted Tomato and Onion Salad (p. 229)
　1 pound dried fusilli
　1/2 pound smoked turkey breast, diced (ask the deli person to cut it thick)
　4 ounces smoked Gouda cheese, diced
　Salt and pepper

1. Make the Roasted Tomato and Onion Salad.
2. Bring a large pot of salted water to a boil and make fusilli according to package directions. Drain.
3. Place the pasta with the turkey, cheese, and Roasted Tomato and Onion Salad in a large bowl and combine ingredients. You should have plenty of sauce, but if it seems too dry, add a little more oil or a splash of wine. Season to taste with salt and pepper, toss, and serve.

Serves 8

Bow-Tie Pasta with Broccoli Rabe

You've seen broccoli rabe in the supermarket: It looks like a head of turnip greens that suddenly decided to sprout tiny little broccoli florets on top. It combines the crunch of broccoli with the bitter pepperiness of other greens. It's too strong to eat raw, but a few minutes of boiling mellows it and turns it into a delightful pasta ingredient. The Italians have used it that way for centuries; now the other side of the Atlantic is catching on. Try it; if you don't like it, feel free to switch to regular broccoli. Pasta is a great way to get your greens, because greens that may seem too bitter on their own actually taste quite good as a contrast to the mildness of the pasta. Anchovies are a great way to add depth of flavor to vegetable or pasta dishes.

1 pound dried bow-tie pasta (farfalle)
2 heads broccoli rabe, chopped, stems removed
1/2 cup olive oil
1 ounce anchovies, drained
2 teaspoons minced garlic
1 teaspoon red pepper flakes (optional)
Salt and pepper
1 cup grated Parmesan cheese

1. Bring a large pot of salted water to a boil. Add the pasta and boil, stirring occasionally, until barely soft (about 12 minutes). After 9 minutes, add the broccoli rabe to the cooking pasta.
2. Drain the pasta and broccoli rabe, reserving 1 cup of the cooking water.
3. Heat the olive oil over medium heat in a skillet large enough to hold the pasta. Add the anchovies, garlic, and red pepper flakes and stir until the anchovies have dissolved and the garlic is golden (about 1 minute).
4. Add the pasta, broccoli rabe, and cooking water, turn the heat to high, and cook, stirring, until the water has disappeared and the sauce is creamy (about 5 minutes). Season with salt and pepper (you might not need any salt because of the anchovies).
5. Sprinkle with Parmesan cheese and serve immediately.

Serves 6

Ravioli in Pumpkin Cream Sauce with Cranberries and Walnuts

Once you've tried this sauce, it will become a weekly staple in your household. All ages love it, it can be made in minutes, and it's high in fiber and vitamin A and low in calories. Keep a couple cans of pumpkin around and you'll always have this on hand as an emergency backup dinner. It's the same idea as the butternut squash sauces some restaurants serve with pasta, only easier. To make it a beautiful and savory holiday dish, sprinkle the top with dried cranberries, toasted walnuts, and a few fresh sage leaves.

1 pound frozen or fresh ravioli or tortellini
1/2 cup walnuts, chopped
1 tablespoon butter
2 tablespoons minced garlic
2 tablespoons fresh sage leaves, minced, or 2 teaspoons dried sage, crumbled
1 15-ounce can pumpkin
1/2 cup milk (additional may be added later to thin sauce)
Salt and pepper
1/4 cup dried cranberries

1. Bring a pot of salted water to a boil and cook the pasta according to the package directions.
2. Meanwhile, heat the oven or toaster oven to 400°F, place the walnuts on a baking sheet, and toast the walnuts until sizzling (about 3 minutes). Set aside.
3. Heat the butter in a large skillet over medium heat until bubbling. Then add the garlic and sauté for 1 minute. Add the sage leaves and sauté an additional 30 seconds. Add the pumpkin and milk and stir.
4. Continue cooking, stirring occasionally, until the sauce is hot and bubbling (about 5 minutes). Thin the sauce to your desired consistency by adding more milk. Season to taste with salt and pepper.
5. Put the cooked pasta in a large serving bowl, cover with the sauce, and sprinkle the top with walnuts and cranberries. Serve at once.

Serves 4 to 6

No-Boil Spinach Lasagne

Admittedly, there's nothing fast about lasagne. It takes a fair amount of prep time, plus an hour to bake. The advantages become apparent when you look at the big picture: It makes a lot, and it's easy to heat in the microwave for lunch the next day. It also freezes beautifully, and it's virtually as easy to make two batches as it is to make one, so double this recipe, freeze the second, and suddenly you're looking at twenty servings of a crowd-pleasing favorite—for a mere hour of work. The invention of noodles that don't need to be boiled cuts down on your workload even more. If you want to be extra decadent, mix a container of pesto sauce into the spinach-cheese mixture.

2 tablespoons olive oil
1 onion, peeled and diced
8 ounces mushrooms, sliced
1 pound ground turkey (or lean ground beef)
1 28-ounce can crushed tomatoes (preferably with Italian seasonings)
1 egg
1 15-ounce container low-fat ricotta cheese
1 pound low-fat mozzarella cheese, grated
1 10-ounce package frozen chopped spinach, thawed, drained, and squeezed dry
Pinch ground nutmeg
1/2 teaspoon salt
8 ounces oven-ready lasagne noodles
1 cup grated Parmesan cheese

1. Heat the olive oil in a large skillet over high heat. Add the onion and mushrooms and sauté until the mushrooms release their liquid.
2. Add the ground turkey and sauté until it changes color (about 3 minutes).
3. Remove skillet from heat and add the crushed tomatoes. Mix well.
4. Preheat the oven to 350°F.
5. Mix the egg, ricotta, mozzarella, spinach, nutmeg, and salt in a large bowl.
6. Spoon just enough of the tomato sauce into a 9x13-inch baking dish to cover the bottom. Cover this with a layer of noodles (three should do it).
7. Spread half the cheese-spinach mixture over the noodles. Cover this with one-third of the remaining tomato sauce.
8. Add another layer of noodles, then the remaining cheese-spinach mixture, then half the remaining tomato sauce.
9. Top with a final layer of noodles, then the remaining tomato sauce, then the Parmesan cheese.
10. Cover with foil and bake in the oven until heated through (about 45 minutes). Remove the foil and bake until the cheese on top is browned (10 to 15 minutes). Let cool for at least 10 minutes before slicing and serving.

Serves 10 to 12

Spicy Peanut Noodles

Peanut or sesame noodles are a staple in many Asian cultures. They've become increasingly popular here, and why not? The creaminess of the sauce makes for a yummy comfort food with more protein and none of the saturated fat of macaroni and cheese. Kids love these, too—though you might have to skip the onions.

The sauce:
2 cups natural peanut butter
1/3 cup white vinegar
1/3 cup soy sauce
2 teaspoons minced garlic
2 tablespoons chili paste or hot sauce
1/3 cup toasted sesame oil
1 cup black tea (or water)

The noodles:
1 pound dried spaghetti
Green onions or cilantro leaves to garnish

1. Place the ingredients for the sauce in a blender or food processor and blend until smooth.
2. Bring a large pot of water to a boil.
3. Add the spaghetti and boil until soft but not mushy (about 8 minutes).
4. Drain the noodles in a colander, put them in a large serving bowl, and top with all the sauce. Garnish and serve.

Serves 6

19. SEAFOOD

Baked Salmon with Apricot Glaze

Shockingly easy, shockingly good.

1/2 cup apricot jam
2 pounds salmon fillets

1 tablespoon canola oil

1. Place a large cast-iron skillet or glass baking dish in the oven and preheat the oven to 400°F.
2. Spread the apricot jam in a thin layer over the top of the salmon fillets.
3. Carefully remove the skillet from the oven, pour in the oil, add the salmon fillets, and bake until the salmon turns pink and flaky (about 7 minutes). Serve immediately.

Serves 6

Grilled Salmon with Wasabi Cream

Wasabi is that spicy green horseradish paste that you get with sushi and that makes your sinuses dial 911. Softening it in a creamy sauce gives you all the flavor benefits without the pain. It pairs beautifully with salmon, which, besides being high in omega-3 fat, is very easy to cook on a grill. If you don't have a grill, you can sear the salmon steaks in a cast-iron skillet over high heat for a similar effect. Wasabi is sold in supermarkets and specialty stores as a powder or as a paste in a tube. The powder is easier to find, but the paste is easier to use and makes for a less grainy cream sauce. This recipe is great with tuna, too.

1/2 cup low-fat sour cream or plain yogurt (or vanilla yogurt for a sweeter sauce)
1 tablespoon wasabi paste or powder
1 teaspoon soy sauce
2 teaspoons canola oil
2 pounds salmon steaks
Salt and pepper

1. Turn the grill to high heat.
2. To make the wasabi cream, spoon the sour cream or yogurt into a small bowl and stir in the wasabi and soy sauce. Taste, and add more wasabi if you like more heat.
3. Brush one teaspoon of oil on one side of the salmon steaks, season with salt and pepper, and place them on the grill, oil side down. Grill for 5 minutes; then brush the top side of the steaks with the remaining oil and flip. Grill for 5 more minutes, then serve with a puddle of the wasabi cream on the side.

Serves 6

Seared Tuna in Olive Sauce

If you've ever eaten sushi, you know that with really fresh fish, the cooking part is optional. This is obvious in the latest restaurant trend: serving tuna that is seared on the outside but rare pink on the inside, like a good steak. An added bonus of this method: Your fish is cooked in 5 minutes! Use only the best quality fish with this recipe. If the tuna steaks are very thick, try slicing them in half lengthwise.

The sauce:
2 tablespoons extra-virgin olive oil
2 ounces green or black olives, pitted and chopped
2 teaspoons capers, drained
1 teaspoon minced garlic

The fish:
Pepper
2 pounds fresh tuna steaks, about 1/2 inch thick
2 tablespoons canola oil

1. Mix the olive oil, olives, capers, and garlic together in a serving bowl. Set aside.
2. Pepper the tuna steaks. (You will not need salt, because the sauce is salty.) Heat the canola oil in a large pan over high heat. Add the tuna and cook until the bottom quarter of an inch turns white (about 2 minutes). Flip and cook the other side until it turns white (about 2 minutes).
3. Serve sauce separately and let each person spoon it on.

Serves 6

Caribbean Coconut Scallops

You may have had coconut shrimp in restaurants. This recipe delivers the same Caribbean-inspired flavors with much less trouble. Unsweetened coconut milk can be found in most supermarkets.

2 tablespoons canola oil (each tablespoon used separately)
2 pounds sea scallops
1 red pepper, seeded and diced
1/2 cup green onions, chopped
2 tablespoons Caribbean seasoning (or Cajun, in a pinch)
1 cup canned unsweetened coconut milk
Juice of 1/2 lime

1. Heat 1 tablespoon of the canola oil in a large nonstick skillet over high heat. Add the scallops and sauté until they turn opaque and then become slightly browned (about 2 minutes). Turn them and sauté on the other side for 1 minute. Remove the scallops from the skillet using a slotted spoon and keep them warm.
2. Add the other tablespoon of oil to the skillet and sauté the red pepper and onions for 1 minute. Sprinkle them with the Caribbean seasoning.
3. Add the coconut milk and cook, stirring occasionally, until it has reduced to the thickness of heavy cream (about 10 minutes). Add the scallops back in and cook just until they are warmed through.
4. Squeeze lime juice over the scallops and serve immediately.

Serves 6

Scallops in Orange Sauce

Scallops are such an ideal weight-loss food that somebody should create the Scallops Diet. Any way you cut it, scallops should become a weekly staple in your home. They are pure protein, delicious, take zero prep time, and cook in minutes. And their natural sweetness lends itself to simple low-calorie sauces, like this Chinese-inspired one. Serve with brown rice and Sesame Green Beans (p. 228) for an Asian-flavored feast.

1 cup orange juice
2 tablespoons soy sauce
1 tablespoon honey
1 teaspoon grated orange peel
3 tablespoons canola oil (1 tablespoon used separately)
2 pounds sea scallops
1 tablespoon minced garlic
Salt and pepper

1. Mix the orange juice, soy sauce, honey, and orange peel in a bowl and set aside.
2. Heat 2 tablespoons of the canola oil in a large nonstick skillet over high heat. Add the scallops and sauté until they turn opaque and then become slightly browned (about 2 minutes). Turn them and sauté on the other side for 1 minute. Remove them with a slotted spoon, transfer to a serving dish, and keep warm.
3. Add the remaining tablespoon of oil to the pan. Add the garlic and sauté until golden (about 30 seconds). Add the orange sauce and boil, stirring frequently, until the sauce has reduced to a syrup (about 5 minutes).
4. Pour the orange sauce over the scallops, adjust seasoning, and serve.

Serves 6

Tuscan Scallops

Tuscan scallops? Well, they may not eat many scallops in Tuscany, but they sure love their white beans! And they'd love this dish. So will you. The beans absorb the scallop flavor and add a creamy sauce of their own (and you use fewer expensive scallops). It's ready in minutes, requires zero prep, and gives you enough protein for an entire day. Serve with a green salad and a glass of white wine for an elegant light dinner.

2 tablespoons extra-virgin olive oil (each tablespoon used separately)	Salt and pepper
1 pound sea scallops	Juice of 1/4 lemon
2 teaspoons minced garlic	2 tablespoons parsley, minced (optional)
1 15-ounce can white beans (preferably cannellini), drained	

1. Heat 1 tablespoon of the oil in a large nonstick skillet over high heat. Add the scallops and garlic and sauté until the scallops turn opaque then become slightly browned (about 2 minutes). Turn them and sauté on the other side for 1 minute.
2. Add the beans and sauté, stirring, until sizzling.
3. Sprinkle with salt, pepper, the remaining tablespoon of olive oil, and lemon juice, and stir together. Garnish with parsley and serve at once.

Serves 4

Crab-Stuffed Portobello Caps

The meatiness of portobello mushrooms—not to mention their huge size—makes them a great meat substitute. When stuffed with crabmeat and Gruyère cheese, they become a fabulous low-carb entrée that will wow company but won't chain you to the kitchen—especially since you can prep the dish hours or even a day in advance and then just do the baking before dinner. If fresh crabmeat is too expensive, substitute canned crab or tuna for a budget version.

4 large portobello mushroom caps, stems removed	1 tablespoon Dijon mustard
1 egg, beaten	1 slice bread, crumbled
6 ounces crabmeat	1/2 teaspoon dried tarragon (optional)
1 tablespoon mayonnaise	4 ounces Gruyère cheese, sliced
1 teaspoon salt	

1. Preheat the oven to 400°F.
2. With oil or nonstick cooking spray, grease a baking dish large enough to fit the 4 mushroom caps.
3. Mix the egg, crabmeat, mayonnaise, salt, mustard, bread, and tarragon (if desired) in a large bowl.
4. Place the mushroom caps gill side up in the baking dish and spread the crabmeat mixture over them.
5. Place in the oven and bake for 20 minutes.
6. Top with the Gruyère slices and bake an additional 5 minutes. Let sit for several minutes before serving.

Serves 4

20. POULTRY

Cashew Chicken Stir-Fry

Nuts are fantastic in stir-fries. Their flavor intensifies, and they add crunch and variety to the dish. Cashews, peanuts, and walnuts all work well. Peanut oil is the best stir-fry oil because it doesn't smoke, even at very high heat. Serve this over brown rice for an easy dinner.

2 tablespoons peanut or canola oil (each tablespoon used separately)
1 pound boneless, skinless chicken breasts, cut into 1/2-inch strips
1 pound broccoli florets, sliced thin

1/2 cup cashews
1 jar stir-fry sauce of your choice

1. Heat 1 tablespoon of the oil in a large nonstick skillet over high heat until quite hot.
2. Add chicken and stir-fry until browned (about 1 minute). Remove chicken to a serving dish.
3. Add the remaining tablespoon of oil to the skillet and stir-fry broccoli about 1 minute. Add cashews and cook an additional 20 seconds.
4. Add stir-fry sauce, return chicken to skillet, stir, and cook until hot and bubbly (about 30 seconds). Serve immediately.

Serves 4

Tandoori Chicken Breasts

Tandoori is a style of cooking in India that involves marinating the meat overnight in a yogurt and spice mixture, then baking it in a special clay oven. The marinating accomplishes two things: The acid in the yogurt tenderizes the meat, and the flavors penetrate all the way through. This recipe is fat-free and works equally well on the grill or in the oven.

3/4 cup plain nonfat yogurt
3 tablespoons curry powder
Juice of 1/4 lemon

1 teaspoon salt
2 pounds boneless, skinless chicken breasts, halved
1/4 cup cilantro, minced (optional)

1. Mix the yogurt, curry powder, lemon juice, and salt together in a large bowl.
2. With a sharp knife, make 3 slits halfway through each chicken breast.
3. Add the chicken breasts to the large bowl and stir to coat them in the yogurt mixture. Make sure the mixture gets inside all the slits. Cover the bowl tightly and allow the chicken to marinate in the refrigerator overnight. (In a pinch, you can get by with just a couple of hours of marinating, but the flavor won't be as good.)
4. When ready to cook, turn the grill on high heat or preheat the oven to 400°F.
5. Bake or grill the chicken breasts. They will take 10 to 12 minutes per side on a grill or 20 minutes in the oven.
6. Garnish with cilantro, if desired, and serve at once.

Serves 6

If you want to stun your dinner guests—and give them something healthy at the same time—serve them mole. Chocolate is not what most people think of as dinner food, but mole is an exception to the rule. And we now know that chocolate is a terrific source of antioxidants. The richness of the chocolate and nuts combines with the dark flavor of the peppers, raisins, and spices to provide a sauce that is like nothing else you've ever tasted. Don't be intimidated by the dried peppers; they are available in every supermarket and are very easy to use. This sauce works well with pork or leftover turkey, too.

The sauce:
4 ounces dried ancho chilies
1/2 cup raisins
1 tablespoon canola oil
2 tablespoons minced garlic
1 onion, peeled and diced
1/2 cup sesame seeds

1/2 cup almonds
1 tablespoon cinnamon
1 tablespoon chili powder
3 ounces dark chocolate, chopped
Salt

1. Stem and seed the chilies. (Don't rub your eyes or touch your face while doing this!) Put them in a large bowl with the raisins, cover with boiling water, and soak for 30 minutes. (Or, to save time, put the chilies, raisins, and water in a small pot and boil for 10 minutes.)
2. Heat the canola oil in a large skillet over high heat. Add the garlic and onion and sauté until the onion is soft (about 2 minutes).
3. Add the sesame seeds, almonds, cinnamon, and chili powder and sauté for 30 seconds. Do not let them burn. Remove the pan from the heat.
4. Drain the chilies and raisins, reserving the liquid. Put them in a food processor with 1/2 cup of the liquid.
5. Add the onion and garlic mixture to the food processor. Process into a paste, adding more of the reserved liquid if necessary. Don't puree; it's nice to leave some texture in the sauce. The paste should be thick.
6. Pour the paste back into the skillet, add the chocolate, and cook, stirring, over low heat until the flavors have married (about 12 minutes). Add salt as needed.

Makes 2 cups paste

The chicken:
1 tablespoon canola oil
2 pounds boneless, skinless chicken breasts

1 cup cilantro, chopped (optional)

1. Heat the canola oil in a large nonstick skillet over high heat.
2. When quite hot, add the chicken breasts. Cook for 4 minutes.
3. Flip the breasts and cook on the other side for 4 minutes.
4. Remove chicken from the pan, slice into strips, and add to the skillet of mole sauce. Heat through until the flavors have married.
5. Sprinkle with cilantro, if desired, and serve over brown rice or with corn or whole-wheat tortillas.

Serves 8

Picadillo is a Latin American dish traditionally made with beef, but ground turkey improves the flavor as well as reducing the saturated fat. Adjust the spices to your liking, but the nuts, raisins, and olives are essential; the salty sweetness gives picadillo its originality. You can serve this over brown rice, accompanied by low-fat yogurt or sour cream and a salad for an easy dinner, or use it as a filling for tortillas. Any way you go, you'll discover a new mainstay in your repertoire.

1 tablespoon canola oil
1 onion, peeled and diced
1 pound ground turkey
1/4 cup water or orange juice
1 tablespoon chili powder
1 tablespoon cinnamon
1/2 cup raisins
1/2 cup almonds, slivered or chopped
1 cup pitted green olives, chopped
Juice of 1/2 lime
Salt and pepper
Cilantro (optional)

1. Heat the canola oil in a large skillet over medium heat. Add the onion and ground turkey and cook, stirring, until the onion turns translucent and the turkey changes color (about 5 minutes).
2. Add the water or juice, chili powder, cinnamon, raisins, almonds, olives, and lime juice and cook until the ingredients have blended and the liquid has reduced by half (about 2 minutes).
3. Season with salt and pepper, garnish with cilantro, if desired, and serve over rice or use to fill tortillas.

Serves 4

Chicken Aloha

You might find this dish in Hawaii. Then again, you might not. In any case, whether you have it for breakfast, lunch, or dinner, it's scrumptious. If you can't get macadamia nuts, cashews work well.

1 cup macadamia nuts
1/2 cup shredded unsweetened coconut
2 tablespoons canola oil
2 pounds boneless, skinless chicken breasts
1 14-ounce can coconut milk
2 cups pineapple, diced
1/4 cup green onions, minced (optional)

1. Preheat the oven to 350°F.
2. Arrange the macadamia nuts and coconut in a single layer on a baking sheet and toast in the oven until golden, shaking the pan periodically (about 5 minutes). Remove from the oven and set aside.
3. Heat the canola oil in a large skillet over high heat.
4. Add the chicken breasts and brown on both sides (about 2 minutes each side).
5. Add the coconut milk to the skillet and simmer over low heat until the chicken is cooked through (about 20 minutes).
6. Add the pineapple and cook for 3 minutes.
7. Serve over brown rice with the macadamia nuts, coconut, and green onions (if desired) sprinkled over the top.

Serves 6

21. MEAT

Beef and Snow Pea Stir-Fry

Stir-fries are an ideal way to learn to cook at home. With a total prep time of less than 10 minutes and a total cooking time of 3 minutes, they can be ready as soon as you get home. (Just have that cooked rice on hand!) Preparing the sauce is the only tricky part, so I recommend using store-bought stir-fry sauce, of which there are many great-tasting varieties. Make sure you get the pan nice and hot with stir-fries so that the ingredients cook quickly and retain all their flavor. Peanut oil works best, because of its high smoking point, but canola does fine, too. Stir-fries are a great way of teaching yourself that a lot of vegetables with smaller amounts of meat taste even better than big hunks of meat by themselves. This recipe uses just snow peas and onions to keep things basic, but you can mix in any vegetables you want: Bell peppers, broccoli, asparagus tips, bok choy (Chinese cabbage), or zucchini would all be good choices. Snow peas are nice because they require next to no prep and are high in vitamins and fiber. Serve this over brown rice for an ultra-easy dinner that will break the meat-and-potatoes rut.

2 tablespoons peanut or canola oil (each tablespoon used separately)
1 pound sirloin, sliced in 1/4-inch-thick strips
1 pound snow peas, trimmed
1 onion, peeled and sliced
1 jar stir-fry sauce of your choice

1. Heat 1 tablespoon of peanut oil in a large nonstick skillet over high heat until quite hot.
2. Add beef and fry, stirring constantly, until browned (about 1 minute). Remove beef to a serving dish.
3. Add the remaining tablespoon of oil to the skillet and stir-fry snow peas and onion about 1 minute.
4. Add stir-fry sauce, return beef to skillet, stir, and cook until hot and bubbly (about 30 seconds). Serve immediately.

Serves 4

Cumin and Orange–Scented Pork Loin

Pork loin has less fat than other cuts of pork. This is surprising, considering how delicious it is. Be sure to trim any fat off the outside and you can relax. Since it contains fewer than 250 calories per serving, this is a very sensible entrée. And with a mere 15 minutes of active prep time, it won't suck up your day, either. Using rubs is an easy way to lock deep flavor into meat. Here, the powdery cumin combines with the olive oil to form a paste that really clings to the pork, browning nicely as it cooks. Once you try this one, you'll want to play around with a variety of rubs for all sorts of meats. And don't forget to toss in some root vegetables (such as Autumn Harvest Medley, p. 229) to cook with the pork. It takes hardly any extra time at all: Presto—dinner's ready!

2 pounds boneless pork loin
2 tablespoons olive oil
1 teaspoon minced garlic
1 tablespoon cumin
1 tablespoon orange juice
1 teaspoon salt
1 teaspoon pepper

1. Preheat the oven to 350°F.
2. Place the pork in a baking pan or on a baking sheet.
3. Combine all ingredients but the pork in a bowl and stir until a paste forms. Using your fingers, rub the paste all over the pork (you don't need to worry about the underside). You can actually do this the morning or night before if you want extra marinating time, though it isn't essential.
4. Roast the pork for about 45 minutes (less for a smaller loin, more for a larger one). It should be crispy on the outside and slightly pink in the center. Let sit 10 minutes before serving.

Serves 6

22. Veggies and Sides

Asparagus Van Gogh

We've all noticed how asparagus spears resemble paintbrushes, so why not take that idea to the next level? There's no better way to break the ice at a dinner party and get everyone in a silly mood than by having the guests paint with their food! (It's also an amazingly effective way to get kids to eat asparagus.) Make sure you cook the asparagus until just tender but still crisp; you don't want mushy paintbrushes. Then use whatever dips will provide an array of different colors, and give your guests a dollop of each color on their plates. They can paint a picture on their plates before using the asparagus brushes to eat the dips. Use at least some store-bought dips to lighten your work load.

2 pounds asparagus, thick ends trimmed

1. Using a vegetable steamer, basket, or colander inside a pot, steam the asparagus spears over 1 inch of boiling water until tender but still crisp (about 3 minutes).
2. Serve the "paintbrushes" on a plate, accompanied by at least 3 different-colored dips.

Serves 4 to 6

Potential dip choices:

- Black: tapenade (olive spread, found with olives in your grocery store)
- Red: roasted red pepper spread (see p. 235)
- Green: pesto (see p. 236) or guacamole (see p. 235)
- Yellow: roasted yellow peppers, pureed; or hollandaise (powdered mix can be found with soups and sauces in your grocery store)
- White: smoked trout spread (found in the fish section of your grocery store)
- Pink: salmon spread (found in the fish or dairy section of your grocery store)
- Blue: good luck!

Zucchini Surprise Fries

How do you make french fries healthy? Easy: Make them out of zucchini instead! These surprise fries are a brilliant way to sneak veggies into kids—and you! Don't skip the salting stage; the salt draws moisture out of the zucchini and collapses air bubbles in them, which keeps the zucchini from soaking up much oil and makes them crisp.

2 medium zucchini, julienned
1 teaspoon salt
1/2 cup canola or peanut oil
2 tablespoons unbleached flour
Salt and pepper

1. Toss the zucchini strips with the salt, set them in a colander in the sink or over a bowl, and drain 20 to 30 minutes. Squeeze any excess moisture out of the zucchini and then press them between paper towels to dry them. If they are too wet, the flour in step 3 won't coat them evenly.
2. Heat the oil in a large skillet until quite hot (but not smoking). Peanut oil is great because its smoking point is so high, but canola works well, too.
3. Toss the zucchini strips with the flour in a large bowl and then add them to the oil, making sure they aren't crowded together. Fry, turning occasionally with a slotted spoon, until they are golden brown (about 5 minutes).
4. Fish out the zucchini with the slotted spoon and drain them on paper towels. Season with salt and pepper and serve immediately.

Serves 2 to 4 (or 1 starving teenager)

Rainbow Pepper Medley

People go to great trouble to roast fresh peppers and peel off their blackened skins to make a tasty appetizer, but all that isn't really necessary. You can save yourself a lot of mess and seared fingertips by using the following method. The result is equally delicious. Most supermarkets now sell bell peppers in rainbow packs of red, yellow, and green, which are perfect for making this dish attractive, though you can use whatever colors appeal to you. Be sure to use extra-virgin olive oil in any dish where the oil will not be cooked; the flavor is far superior to other oils.

    4 bell peppers of varying colors
    1/4 cup extra-virgin olive oil
    1 teaspoon minced garlic
    Salt and pepper

1. Slice the peppers in half and remove the stems, seeds, and any inner membranes. Cut the peppers into strips.
2. Place the peppers in a large skillet that can be covered. Add about 1/2 inch of water, cover, and bring to a simmer.
3. Cook until the peppers are tender but not mushy (about 10 minutes).
4. Drain the peppers, put them in a large bowl, add the oil, garlic, salt, and pepper; then toss. Serve immediately or at room temperature.

Serves 6 as an appetizer or side dish

Sesame Green Beans

So easy, so versatile, and so delicious! Make them spicy by adding hot sauce or chili peppers if you like.

    2 pounds green beans, trimmed
    1/4 cup extra-virgin olive oil
    2 tablespoons toasted sesame oil
    Salt to taste

1. Bring a large pot of salted water to a boil.
2. Add green beans and cook until tender but still crisp (5 to 6 minutes). Drain.
3. Place the beans in a large bowl, add the olive and sesame oil, and toss. Correct seasoning and add more olive oil if they seem too dry. Serve immediately or at room temperature.

Serves 6

Roasted Tomato and Onion Salad

Roasting vegetables brings out their sweetness, which makes this a great way to use store-bought tomatoes that aren't very sweet. Of course, it only gets better if you use ripened summer tomatoes. Sprinkle bread crumbs over the top if you want a little golden crust.

2 pounds tomatoes, halved
1 pound onions (preferably Vidalia or another
    sweet variety), peeled and quartered
1/4 cup extra-virgin olive oil

1 teaspoon dried oregano
1 teaspoon salt
1 tablespoon red-wine vinegar

1. Preheat the oven to 450°F.
2. Place the tomatoes and onions in a large bowl. Add half the olive oil, the oregano, and the salt; then toss.
3. Place the tomatoes (cut side up) and the onions in a baking dish and roast until wrinkled and starting to blacken (about 20 minutes).
4. Put the tomatoes and onions in a serving dish, toss with the remaining olive oil and the vinegar, adjust seasoning, and serve.

Serves 8

Autumn Harvest Medley

When the autumn chill first arrives and the carrots, parsnips, and onions are grown and plump in the ground, it's the perfect time to warm the house up with a roasting oven and warm yourself up with some subtly sweet root vegetables. If you haven't had parsnips in a long time, this is your chance! They have a natural buttery sweetness and taste like nothing else. The best time to make this dish is when you'll be roasting something else in the oven, like a chicken or my Cumin and Orange–Scented Pork Loin (p. 225), because your time commitment will be minimal.

1 pound carrots, trimmed, peeled, and chopped
1 pound parsnips, trimmed, peeled, and chopped
2 large onions, peeled and quartered
1/4 cup olive oil

1 teaspoon cinnamon
1 teaspoon salt
1 teaspoon pepper

1. Preheat the oven to 400°F.
2. Place the carrots, parsnips, and onions in a large bowl, drizzle the olive oil over them, and stir to coat them. Season with the cinnamon, salt, and pepper.
3. Place the root veggies one layer deep in a baking pan and bake until they are tender and starting to brown (about 1 hour).

Serves 8

Butternut Squash with Tarragon

Tarragon is an herb that doesn't get enough attention. Called "the little dragon" in France, it improves almost everything, from chicken and fish to vegetables. It may be at its finest with winter squash, where it makes their sweet, mild flavors richer and sharper. At first, you may think the tarragon hasn't added much flavor, but after the dish has sat for 10 or 15 minutes, the heat and moisture of the squash will draw the aromatic oils out of the tarragon leaves. You'll love the result. You'll also love cooking this in the microwave—no cleanup! (If using a conventional oven, roast the squash for 1 hour at 400°F.) Try this at Thanksgiving, using your favorite winter squash.

1 butternut squash (about 2 pounds), halved   2 tablespoons minced fresh tarragon, or 2 teaspoons dried
2 tablespoons butter   Salt and pepper

1. Place the squash cut-side-down on a microwave-safe plate or glass dish with a little water in the bottom. Microwave on high for 10 minutes. Check the squash. If it isn't soft enough, microwave for an additional 2 minutes.
2. Scrape the seeds out of the squash and discard, then scrape all the flesh into a serving bowl.
3. Stir in the butter and tarragon and let sit at least 5 minutes for the flavors to come out. Season with salt and pepper and serve.

Serves 8

Garlicky Cauliflower Mash

Everybody is mashing cauliflower these days. It makes a brilliant low-carb substitute for mashed potatoes. You can fool a lot of people! However, it usually takes butter and cream to do so. But cauliflower lends itself well to a number of spices, so forget trying to fool people and let cauliflower be cauliflower. This recipe gives you two options: mashed potato–style with butter and cream, or delectable Italian-style with olive oil and garlic.

1 head cauliflower, chopped, or 12 ounces cauliflower florets   2 tablespoons minced garlic (optional)
1/4 cup milk or cream   Salt and pepper
3 tablespoons butter or olive oil

1. Place the cauliflower in a pot of salted water and boil until very soft (15 to 20 minutes). Remember, you want it to mash very easily.
2. Drain the cauliflower and put it in a food processor. (You can mash it by hand, but you won't get that whipped potatolike consistency.) For the mashed potato–style, add the butter, milk or cream, as well as some salt and pepper. For the Italian-style, add the olive oil, the garlic, and some salt and pepper. Blend until very smooth. Adjust seasoning and serve.

Serves 4

Spinach with Roasted Garlic Cream

This is a fancy way of disguising good old creamed spinach and making it fit for company. (And because of the heavy cream, you might want to reserve this dish for such an occasion.) In truth, creamed spinach can be really good, because spinach and cream have such a natural affinity. The earthy flavor of roasted garlic and the color of red peppers make it new again! (This also makes an excellent omelette filling; see omelette instructions on p. 194.) You can roast your own garlic in the oven, but you'll save yourself half an hour by using the kind that comes in a jar. (And why not use that half hour for a nice walk?)

1 10-ounce package frozen chopped spinach, thawed and squeezed dry
1/4 cup heavy cream
1 tablespoon minced roasted garlic
1/4 teaspoon nutmeg
Salt and pepper
1 roasted red pepper, diced (optional)

1. Combine the spinach, cream, garlic, and nutmeg in a large skillet. Add salt and pepper to taste. Then cook over medium heat until the spinach is wilted and the sauce is bubbling. Mix in the red pepper. Correct seasoning and serve as a side dish.

Serves 4 to 6

Southwest Black Bean Fritters

These fritters are equally good as a high-protein breakfast, a side dish, or a meatless dinner. And with the contrasting colors of the toppings, they are plenty fancy for company.

Fritters:
1 15-ounce can black beans, drained
1 egg
2 tablespoons yellow cornmeal or whole-wheat flour
1/2 teaspoon cayenne (optional)
1/2 teaspoon salt
1/4 cup frozen corn kernels, thawed
1/2 red bell pepper, stemmed, seeded, and diced
2 tablespoons minced onion
2 tablespoons canola oil

Toppings:
Low-fat sour cream
Salsa or roasted red peppers
Avocado or green onions

1. Puree the beans in a food processor. Add the egg, cornmeal, cayenne (if desired), and salt; then pulse until combined.
2. Scoop the bean mixture into a large bowl and mix in the corn kernels, red bell pepper, and onion.
3. Form the fritters into patties, as you would hamburger, and arrange them on a plate near the stove.
4. Heat the canola oil in a large nonstick skillet over high heat. Fill the pan with fritters, leaving enough room so they don't touch. Flatten the fritters by pressing on them with a spatula, then fry until they are brown and crispy on the bottom (about 5 minutes). Flip and fry on the other side for 3 minutes.
5. Drain the fritters on paper towels. Serve at once, topped with a dollop of sour cream, a splash of salsa or some roasted red peppers, and a sprinkling of avocado or green onion.

Serves 2 to 4

Cajun Red Beans and Rice

It's almost embarrassing how easy this recipe is! It shouldn't taste this good . . . but it does! So who's complaining? For extra authenticity, sauté onions and celery in canola oil and mix them in at the end.

1 cup brown rice
2 1/2 cups water
1 tablespoon Cajun or blackened seasoning
1 15-ounce can red kidney beans, drained
4 ounces ham, diced (optional)

1. Combine the rice, water, Cajun seasoning, and red beans in a pot. Bring to a boil.
2. Immediately lower the heat as much as possible and simmer, covered, stirring occasionally, until all the water is absorbed (about 45 minutes).
3. Stir in the ham, if desired, and serve as a side dish.

Serves 8

Coconut Rice

Here's an easy way to add a tropical accent to dinner. This side dish goes wonderfully with many entrées in this book, especially Chicken Aloha, Baked Salmon with Apricot Glaze, or Tandoori Chicken Breasts. For extra protein, throw a can of drained black beans into the rice.

1 cup brown rice
1 14-ounce can unsweetened light coconut milk
3/4 cup water
1/2 teaspoon salt
1/4 cup cilantro, minced (optional)

Combine rice, coconut milk, water, and salt in a pot and cover. Bring to a boil; then immediately reduce the heat to as low a setting as possible. Simmer until all the liquid has been absorbed (about 45 minutes). Stir and serve, garnished with cilantro if desired.

Serves 6

No-Fail Brown Rice

For anyone still suspicious of brown rice, here is the solution. Nothing could be simpler! Make this traditional brown rice when you can, and keep a package of instant brown rice on hand for when you've got only 10 minutes. (For richer flavor, substitute chicken or vegetable broth for half the water.)

1 cup brown rice
2 1/2 cups water
1/2 teaspoon salt

1. In a large pot, combine the rice, water, and salt. Stir and then cover.
2. Bring the rice to a boil. Immediately lower the heat as low as possible and simmer, covered, until all the water has been absorbed (about 45 minutes). Let sit for a minute; then fluff with a fork and serve.

Makes 3 1/2 cups; serves 6

23. SNACKS AND APPETIZERS

Roasted Red Pepper Spread

This traditional dip from the Middle East is yet another great substitute for the typical store-bought high-fat, low-nutrition sour cream–based dips we tend to use. It's a perfect example of the philosophy that eating healthy doesn't mean sacrifice; it means better food, too! Serve with crackers, pita chips, or crusty bread. (Look for crackers that are made from whole grains and are free of transfats.)

1 jar roasted red peppers, drained
1 cup walnuts or almonds
2 tablespoons extra-virgin olive oil
Juice of 1/4 lemon
1 teaspoon honey
1 teaspoon cumin
1/2 teaspoon salt

Combine all the ingredients in a food processor or blender and blend until smooth.

Makes 3 cups

Guacamole

The secret of good guacamole is to use really ripe avocados. They should be nice and soft. If you have that, you don't need to do much at all. A little salt, a little lime juice, and you have the world's perfect good-fat appetizer and condiment.

2 ripe avocados, peeled and pitted
Juice of 1/2 lime
1/2 teaspoon salt
1 teaspoon chili powder
1 tablespoon salsa (optional)
1/4 ripe tomato, diced (optional)

1. Place the avocado, lime juice, salt, and chili powder in a large bowl and mash. Stir in the salsa or tomato (if desired). Serve with whole-grain tortilla chips.

Serves 4 as an appetizer

We're all used to seeing pesto as a pasta sauce in Italian restaurants, but its potential uses go well beyond that. Pesto's explosion of flavor makes it the perfect dip for raw veggies. Substitute it for mayonnaise on your favorite sandwich. Or use it as a sauce for grilled zucchini or steamed green beans. Healthwise, pesto gives you a great one-two combo of good fats from the olive oil and nuts, plus lots of vitamins and antioxidants in the basil and garlic. This recipe substitutes walnuts for the traditional pine nuts to take advantage of walnuts' omega-3 content, but you can use any nut or seed you like. This also changes the ratio of nuts to cheese to keep the saturated fat to a minimum.

2 cups tightly packed fresh basil leaves
2 cloves garlic, chopped
1/2 cup walnuts
1/2 teaspoon salt
1/4 cup grated Parmesan cheese
3/4 cup extra-virgin olive oil

1. Place the basil, garlic, walnuts, salt, and cheese in a food processor. Process until finely minced but not pureed (pesto is better if it retains a little texture).
2. Add the olive oil and process to desired consistency. Store in an airtight jar in the refrigerator for up to 1 week.

Makes 3 1/2 cups, enough for 8 pasta servings

No one ever claimed spanakopita was healthy, but we all agree it's delicious. Fortunately, you can get all the deliciousness without any of the butter with these delightful snacks. Once on hand, they work equally well for a quickly microwaved breakfast, a midmorning lift, or cut up into small squares and served on toothpicks for brunch or hors d'oeuvres. The eggs add lots of protein, the spinach and whole-wheat flour contribute vitamins and fiber, and the carb content is quite low. If you don't like the tang of feta cheese, feel free to substitute your favorite.

1 10-ounce package frozen chopped spinach, thawed and squeezed dry
3 eggs, beaten
8 ounces feta cheese, crumbled
3 tablespoons whole-wheat flour
1/2 teaspoon salt
1/4 teaspoon grated nutmeg
4 ounces grated Parmesan cheese

1. Preheat the oven to 350°F.
2. Grease an 8x8-inch baking pan or use nonstick cooking spray.
3. Mix together the spinach, eggs, feta, flour, salt, and nutmeg in a large bowl. Pour this mixture into the baking pan.
4. Sprinkle the Parmesan cheese over the top and bake 25 to 30 minutes, until the cheese on top is golden brown and bubbly and a knife stuck in the middle comes out clean. Remove from the oven and let cool at least 10 minutes before slicing. Serve hot or at room temperature.

Makes approximately 16 2-inch squares

Cashew-Ginger Trail Mix

This is almost too easy to qualify as a recipe. It's more of an idea, but new ideas can make a big difference in your diet. If you get bored eating plain nuts for your snacks, liven things up with trail mixes. Their mixture of protein, good fat, fiber, and carbs will give you energy with staying power to keep you at peak performance, whether it's on the trail or in the office. Use crystallized ginger to take advantage of ginger's many healing qualities. You can also come up with any combination of nuts and dried fruit that works for you.

2 ounces roasted cashews
1 ounce crystallized ginger pieces

Mix the cashews and ginger in a small bowl.

Serves 1

Here are some other combinations you might try:

- Peanuts, raisins, and chocolate chips
- Almonds and dried figs
- Macadamia nuts, dried pineapple, and dried banana chips
- Walnuts and dried apricots

Spicy Tamari Almonds

An excellent way to liven up plain almonds. Warning: These are addictive!

1 pound almonds
2 tablespoons tamari or soy sauce
1/4 teaspoon cayenne (optional)

1. Preheat the oven to 375°F.
2. Spread the almonds one layer deep on a baking sheet, sprinkle with the cayenne (if desired), and bake until sizzling (about 15 minutes).
3. Pour the almonds into a large bowl, sprinkle the tamari or soy sauce over them, and stir to coat. Spread the almonds back on the baking sheet and allow them to cool to room temperature. They will store in an airtight container for at least a month.

Makes 1 pound

24. DESSERTS

Guava Granita

Granitas are the simplest, healthiest desserts possible: just semifrozen fruit juice crushed into jagged slivers and served in elegant wine or martini glasses. When done right, the little fruit crystals burst in your mouth, releasing surprising flavor. The trick is to get the texture right by scoring the ice with a fork periodically so no lumps form and it doesn't freeze into one solid sheet. You want as many crystals as possible. You can use any fruit juice you like, but because you eat so little of this at a time, it needs to be sweeter than you think. Use a sweet tropical juice like guava, mango, or pineapple (you can often find cans of these in the international section of supermarkets); apple cider; or sweetened citrus or berry juices. Adding a pinch of salt also helps bring out the fruit flavor of the juice.

Pinch of salt (optional)
Sugar (optional)
2 cups guava juice
Mint leaves for garnish

1. Stir the salt (and sugar if you need extra sweetness) into the juice and pour the juice into a pan wide enough that the juice will be only about 1 inch deep. Cover the pan with plastic wrap and place in the freezer for 30 to 60 minutes, until the juice just begins to freeze.
2. Score the liquid with a fork to make uneven crystals; then return it to the freezer. Score it again every 30 minutes until completely frozen (usually takes 2 to 3 hours).
3. Spoon the crystals into wide-mouthed wine or martini glasses or small bowls, garnish with mint leaves, and serve with spoons.

Serves 4

Lemon Almond Cookies

What do you say to a cookie with no flour and no butter or oil? How about "Hello, dessert!" This is the simplest cookie recipe you'll ever find, and certainly the healthiest. Just almonds, lemon juice, and sugar. The trick is to grind the almonds very fine, so they act like regular flour.

Butter or oil for greasing cookie sheet
2 1/2 cups almonds
1 cup sugar
2 teaspoons lemon juice
2 teaspoons almond extract

1. Grease a cookie sheet with the butter or oil.
2. Put the almonds, sugar, lemon juice, and almond extract in a food processor and chop until the almonds are very fine and a dough has formed.
3. Pick up handfuls of dough, squeeze them tightly into 1-inch patties, and place them on the cookie sheet. Let the cookies sit at room temperature for at least 2 hours. This helps to keep them from falling apart.
4. Preheat the oven to 375°F.
5. Bake for 8 to 10 minutes until the cookies are golden brown. Remove from the oven and let cool on a rack or on brown paper bags.

Makes about 30 small cookies

Oatmeal-Raisin Chocolate Chip Cookies

These cookies have so much going for them—the fiber, the vitamins, the antioxidants—that you don't need to hesitate before eating them. They make an excellent snack—and a decent breakfast, too! As a variation, substitute 1/2 cup finely chopped crystallized ginger for the raisins.

    1 cup whole-wheat flour
    1 1/2 cups old-fashioned oats
    1/2 teaspoon baking powder
    1/4 teaspoon baking soda
    1/2 teaspoon salt
    1/2 teaspoon cinnamon
    1 egg
    1 stick butter, softened
    1 teaspoon vanilla extract
    3/4 cup sugar
    1/2 cup raisins
    1/2 cup chocolate chips

1. Preheat the oven to 350°F. Grease two cookie sheets.
2. In a large bowl, mix together the dry ingredients (the flour, oats, baking powder, baking soda, salt, and cinnamon).
3. Cream the wet ingredients (the egg, butter, vanilla, and sugar) in a separate bowl or in a food processor.
4. Pour the dry ingredients into the wet ones and mix until smooth. Fold in the raisins and chocolate chips.
5. Drop heaping tablespoonfuls of batter onto the greased cookie sheets, about an inch apart from one another. Bake in the oven until the cookies are browned (8 to 10 minutes). Remove them from the oven and let cool on a rack or on brown paper bags.

Makes about 36 small cookies

Sugar-Free Apple Pie

Artificial sweeteners don't always work well in desserts, because sugar adds a wonderful moistness and flavor to baked goods that can't be matched. With fruit desserts, however, artificial sweeteners work fine. Splenda is an artificial sweetener with a strong safety record and a taste indistinguishable from sugar, so it's the one used in this recipe and the one that follows. This apple pie has about a third fewer calories than a normal pie, and far fewer carbs. The danger, however, is that you'll think you can eat as much as you want because it's "sugar-free." Sorry, one piece only!

1 package refrigerated piecrust (contains 2 crusts)
8 medium pie apples, such as Macintosh, peeled, cored, and sliced
2 tablespoons unbleached flour
1/2 cup Splenda no-calorie sweetener
Juice of 1/4 lemon
1 teaspoon cinnamon
1/4 teaspoon salt

1. Preheat the oven to 400°F. Allow the piecrusts to come to room temperature.
2. Unfold the piecrusts and press one crust into the bottom of a 9-inch pie pan. It should overhang the edge slightly.
3. Mix the apples, flour, Splenda, lemon juice, cinnamon, and salt in a large bowl. Pour the mixture into the crust in the pie pan.
4. Cover the pie with the remaining piecrust. Use a fork to seal the edges together by crimping all the way around. Cut off any leftover crust, prick the top with the fork here and there to allow steam to escape, and place the pie in the oven.
5. Bake for about 40 to 45 minutes, or until the top is golden brown. Before serving, let cool for at least 30 minutes so that the filling thickens.

Makes about 12 small slices

Sugar-Free Pumpkin Pie

Since pumpkin pie already has lots of moistness and texture from the pumpkin, it's a perfect candidate for going sugar-free.

1 frozen piecrust in a pie tin
3 eggs, beaten
1 15-ounce can pumpkin
1 10-ounce can evaporated milk
1 cup Splenda no-calorie sweetener

1 teaspoon vanilla extract
2 teaspoons cinnamon
1/2 teaspoon nutmeg
1/2 teaspoon ground clove
1/2 teaspoon salt

1. Preheat the oven to 375°F.
2. Put the piecrust in the oven and bake until golden brown (10 to 15 minutes).
3. Meanwhile, mix the rest of the ingredients together in a large bowl.
4. When the crust is ready, remove it from the oven, pour the pumpkin mixture into it, and bake the pie in the oven until the center is set (about 45 minutes). Let cool completely before serving.

Makes about 12 small slices

Pears Poached in Wine Sauce

This French classic is a good way to make dessert exciting without using massive quantities of sugar (and it contains no fat). You may have had poached pears in a restaurant and assumed they were hard to make. You were wrong!

2 cups red wine
1 cup sugar
1/4 cup orange juice or Grand Marnier
1 teaspoon orange zest (optional)
1 cinnamon stick
6 ripe but firm pears, peeled and cored

1. Combine all ingredients but the pears in a pan large enough to fit the pears and bring to a boil. Cook over low heat, stirring, until the sugar dissolves (about 5 minutes).
2. Add the pears, cover the pan, and poach, turning them occasionally, until they are soft (about 8 minutes). Turn off the heat and let the pears cool in the syrup. You'll need to turn them every so often if you want the wine color to spread evenly.
3. To serve, stand the pears up on individual plates or bowls and drizzle with the syrup.

Serves 6

Broiled Grapefruit with Cinnamon

Here's another way to eat a scrumptious, guilt-free dessert!

2 grapefruits, halved
2 tablespoons brown sugar
1 tablespoon cinnamon

1. Preheat the broiler.
2. Using a serrated knife, section the grapefruit but leave it in the rind. Place the grapefruit halves cut side up in a baking dish.
3. Mix the brown sugar and cinnamon in a small bowl, then sprinkle this evenly over the 4 grapefruit halves.
4. Place the dish under the broiler and cook until the sugary topping begins to bubble (about 4 minutes). Serve at once.

Serves 4

Chocolate Fondue with Fresh Fruit

Dark chocolate is rich in antioxidants, whose health benefits make up for chocolate's high fat content. When melted in canola oil to create a luscious fondue, it makes a dessert that is indulgent yet perfectly healthy—especially when paired with fresh fruit. Indulge infrequently, please.

2 tablespoons canola oil
8 ounces dark chocolate (not baking), broken into pieces
1 tablespoon vanilla extract
2 to 4 pounds fresh fruit of your choice, peeled if needed and cut in mouth-size pieces for dipping (Try strawberries, bananas, orange sections, pineapple chunks, and mango or peach slices.)

1. Heat the oil in a small saucepan over low heat. Add the chocolate and stir until melted. Then add the vanilla and stir.
2. Pour the fondue into a serving dish and serve accompanied by fresh fruit and forks for dipping the fruit.

Serves 8

25. BEVERAGES

Peachy Green Tea Punch

A number of recent studies have shown that green tea may have important cancer-fighting properties. If you've never tried green tea, this punch is a great way to get started. Drink this hot or cold. You'll find that you need only a hint of sweetness in your drinks if there are other interesting flavors, as well.

4 bags green tea
2 bags peach-flavored herbal tea
1 bag mint tea
1/4 cup honey or sugar

1. Bring about 2 cups of water to a boil in a kettle.
2. Place the tea bags into a teapot and pour the boiling water over them. Brew for 5 minutes and then remove tea bags.
3. Mix in the honey or sugar while the liquid is still hot and then stir.
4. Fill a pitcher with 4 cups cold water and pour the tea into it. Taste and add more cold water if it is too strong.

Makes 6 to 8 cups, depending on strength

Holiday Spice Tea

When snow is on the ground and carols are in the air, nothing tastes better than steaming mugs of this classic winter treat.

1 orange
4 bags black tea
2 cinnamon sticks
1/4 cup sugar

1. Fill a kettle full of water and bring to a boil.
2. Peel the orange, reserving the peel.
3. Place the tea bags, orange peel, and cinnamon sticks in a teapot. Fill the pot with boiling water and brew for 5 minutes. After stirring, remove the tea bags, cinnamon sticks, and orange peel.
4. Juice the orange and add this liquid to the tea, along with the sugar. Taste, adjust for sweetness, and serve.

Makes 4 cups

Appendix A

TEN FOOD DEVELOPMENTS THAT WILL IMPROVE YOUR LIFE

Eating foods in their natural form doesn't have to mean hours of prep time. More and more, companies are recognizing that our desire to eat healthy foods is often derailed by time constraints, and they are giving us some very handy new options. Here are my ten current favorites. All are widely available in supermarkets. You may already use some of them, but try out the others and see if they help make eating well a cinch.

1. Bagged Broccoli and Cauliflower Florets

These fresh delights come in twelve-ounce bags. There is no washing, no chopping, and no waste. You can even cook them right in the bag! Just open one side, pop it in the microwave on high for four to five minutes, and serve. You can steam them even faster. Of course, broccoli and cauliflower are also delicious raw, so take a bag to work with a healthy dip for a vitamin-rich, utensil-free snack. With these around, there's no reason to use frozen broccoli, which takes longer to cook and has a less appealing texture.

2. Baby Carrots

If you're a parent, you're already familiar with the official snack of America's children. Don't be fooled by the "baby" part; baby spinach may consist of young leaves, but baby carrots are regular grown-up carrots that have been peeled and chopped down to bite size. Still, who cares? A carrot is a carrot, and these are another ready-to-eat snack that beats the heck out of chips.

3. Bagged Greens

If you have any doubt that bagged greens are one of the phenomenal food successes of the past decade, just look at how much real estate they take up in supermarkets now. Somebody is buying all those greens, and likely it's you. Let the purists complain about how much more the greens cost per ounce; I know that if I don't have to wash, dry, and chop my lettuce, I'm a lot more likely to eat it. The extra cents are a great investment in my health—and sanity. And the variety of greens makes a much more interesting salad than plain lettuce.

4. Cubed Butternut Squash

Food companies have finally realized that those big rock-hard winter squashes are intimidating to people. How am I gonna cut through that thing? And what do I do with it? It's actually not that complicated—see my Butternut Squash with Tarragon recipe (p. 230) to learn to work with squash in its natural state, but if the packaged cubes make you eat more vitamin A–rich squash, they're well worth it. Just steam or microwave them for a few minutes and they'll be ready to eat.

5. Minced Garlic

The purists have a point when it comes to garlic. The minced garlic that comes in jars *doesn't* taste the same as raw cloves—not as much fire—but if ease of use is a key factor for you, go with the jars. You just scoop what you need into your dish and don't have to bother with knives, garlic presses, or cleanup. The labels on these jars claim that half a teaspoon of minced garlic is the equivalent of one raw clove, but I think a full teaspoon is closer. One nice product that's starting to appear is minced roasted garlic. That's a flavor I could eat every day!

6. Instant Brown Rice

Most people like the taste of brown rice but not the hour of cooking it requires. Fortunately, there are now several varieties of instant brown rice on the market. There goes the last excuse people had not to cook brown rice. Instant brown rice needs only five minutes in boiling water. It's regular brown rice that's been precooked and then dried. It may not taste quite as good, but all the important fiber is still there.

7. Oven-Ready Lasagne Noodles

Lasagne is a dish people make only once a year because of the mess and trouble involved. But the prep time has been cut in half by the introduction of oven-ready lasagne noodles. No more boiling the noodles, then fishing the slippery things out of the pot and trying to deal with them without burning your fingers or ripping the noodles. Now it's just mix your cheese sauce, open your tomato sauce, and layer these with noodles straight out of the box. Nice!

8. Protein Bars

It used to be that all snack options in the store were unhealthy. That's changing fast. With our new interest in health, companies are rushing to provide us with a wide choice of bars that offer a healthy mix of whole grains and protein from nuts or soy flour. For breakfast or a snack, they are one more great way to squeeze junk-food habits out of your life.

9. Healthy Frozen Dinners

A style of "healthy" frozen dinner came out in the nineties, but it did nobody any favors. Those dinners were very low in fat but very high in carbs, usually from pasta and sugar, and they did little more than make you even hungrier two hours after you ate them. Now there are some much better options on the scene. Look for dinners fairly low in carbs and saturated fat but full of vegetables. One unexpected benefit of frozen dinners is that they often come in single servings, so there's no temptation to dip back for more! In addition, these dinners tend to range from 220 to 320 calories, which isn't all that much. Serve with a side salad for a satisfying meal.

10. Triscuit

Triscuit? Triscuit isn't new. No, but it's now transfat-free! And it's always been made from 100 percent whole grain, making it sound suspiciously like health food. We get so used to seeing the endless list of unpronounceable ingredients in our food products that it can come as a shock to look at the side of a Triscuit box and see only four ingredients: whole wheat, soybean oil, salt, and monoglycerides (naturally occurring fatty acids that improve shelf life). Triscuits aren't low in calories, so don't eat a whole box, but a few served with something useful, like smoked fish, sliced turkey, or Roasted Red Pepper Spread (p. 235), makes a very sensible snack.

Now that the whistle has been blown on transfats, many companies are scrambling to get away from them as fast as they can. By the time you read this, half the crackers, cookies, and chips in America will be transfat-free. Check a box of your favorites. If they don't list transfats in the nutrition info with a big fat goose egg next to it, pick a new favorite.

Appendix B
TEN SUPERFOODS

Almost all natural foods are good for you in various ways, but some are such nutritional superstars that they belong in a category all their own. I call them SUPERFOODS! The following ten superfoods are featured in many of the recipes in this book, but I group them here as well to give you a ready reference. If you want a quick self-check of how you're doing dietwise, look here. If these ten foods are making regular appearances in your diet, you're doing pretty well! If not, use the recipes and suggestions in this book to figure out ways to incorporate as many of the ten as possible.

Tomatoes
- Excellent source of vitamin C and the antioxidant lycopene
- Good source of vitamin A
- Very low in calories
- May help prevent prostate cancer

Suggested Recipes
Roasted Tomato and Onion Salad (p. 229)
No-Boil Spinach Lasagne (p. 213)

Salmon
- Excellent source of protein, calcium, tryptophan, vitamin D, B vitamins, phosphorus, magnesium, and selenium
- Rich in omega-3 and other good fats
- Reduces cholesterol and protects against heart disease

Suggested Recipes
Baked Salmon with Apricot Glaze (p. 215)
Grilled Salmon with Wasabi Cream (p. 215)
Scrambled Eggs with Smoked Salmon (p. 192)
Smoky Fish Chowder (p. 209)

Green Tea
- Zero-calorie drink!
- Excellent source of flavonoid antioxidants
- May help prevent heart disease and some cancers
- May slow aging

Suggested Recipes
Peachy Green Tea Punch (p. 245)

Broccoli

- Excellent source of fiber, folate, vitamins A and C
- Good source of antioxidants and many minerals and vitamins
- May help prevent many cancers and heart disease
- Very low in calories

Suggested Recipes

Garden of Eden Pasta Salad (p. 201)
Bow-Tie Pasta with Broccoli Rabe (p. 211)

Apples

- Excellent source of pectin and fiber
- Low in calories
- The best source of quercetin, which protects against Alzheimer's disease

Suggested Recipes

Sugar-Free Apple Pie (p. 242)

Spinach

- Excellent source of folate, vitamins A and K, manganese, and magnesium
- Good source of calcium, potassium, B vitamins, vitamin C, and fiber
- High in antioxidants that prevent eye diseases and cancer
- Very low in calories

Suggested Recipes

Spinach and Chèvre Omelette (p. 194)
Wilted Spinach Salad with Bacon (p. 200)
No-Boil Spinach Lasagne (p. 213)
Spinach with Roasted Garlic Cream (p. 231)
Spinach-Feta Bites (p. 237)

Walnuts

- Excellent source of vitamin E, healthy fats, and fiber
- Good source of protein, manganese, copper, and tryptophan
- The best non-animal source of omega-3 fat
- May help prevent heart disease and stroke

Cinnamon-Walnut Muffins (p. 190)
Turkey Pesto Wrap (p. 195)
Linguine with Pesto (p. 210)
Ravioli in Pumpkin Cream Sauce with Cranberries and Walnuts (p. 212)

Oats
- Excellent source of fiber
- Good source of manganese and selenium
- Contain unique antioxidants that help prevent heart disease
- Reduce cholesterol

Suggested Recipes
Cranberry-Almond Granola (p. 190)
Oatmeal-Raisin Chocolate Chip Cookies (p. 241)

Blueberries
- Excellent source of flavonoid antioxidants
- Good source of fiber and vitamin C
- May help prevent heart disease and stroke
- May slow aging

Suggested Recipes
Blueberry Breakfast Smoothie (p. 189)

Garlic
- The best source of the antioxidant allicin
- Reduces cholesterol and blood pressure
- May help prevent heart disease and cancer

Suggested Recipes
Half the recipes in this book!

Recipe Index

Get in Touch with Me

If you get in shape by using the plan in this book, I'd love to hear your story! Even if you just have some basic questions about nutrition or exercise, or want to follow one of my Walk Diets on-line, I encourage you to contact me. The best way to get in touch is to visit my Web site:

WWW.LESLIESANSONE.COM

There, you'll find a wealth of information about healthy eating, exercising, and living. You'll also find a community of caring people sharing their advice on how to keep mind, body, and spirit healthy. I welcome you to join the conversation!

Want to keep walking with Leslie?

Join the club!

Leslie Sansone's Walk Club makes you part of the fun every day of the year. It's the perfect way to keep your energy high and get the support you need to stick to your new walking and eating goals. With a membership in the club, you get these fantastic features:

- An all-new Walk Diet every month! Let Leslie be your personal trainer with daily workout routines, Walk Talks that remind you of the health benefits you achieve while you exercise, and Walk Boosters to take your weight loss to the next level.
- Your very own online Walk Log. Keep a permanent record of your success that you can access from any computer and print out.
- Walk Right Now streaming video. Forgot your DVD? You can view a workout with Leslie right on any computer, any time.
- Live auditoriums. Each week gives you a chance to ask Leslie or a special guest any question you want.
- Bulletin board. Meet others like you who are on the same program. Ask questions. Find local walk buddies. Get or give advice.
- A 15 percent discount on all products! And special offers exclusively for Walk Club members!

An exclusive offer for purchasers of *Eat Smart, Walk Strong:*

Get a FREE 12-Week Membership in Leslie's Walk Club!

Go to www.LeslieSansone.com/eatsmart/walkstrong to join the Walk Club

We can't wait to meet you!

offer good until January 1, 2008